THE URBAN HEALTH CRISIS

Strategies for health for all in the face of rapid urbanization

**Report of the Technical Discussions
at the Forty-fourth World Health Assembly**

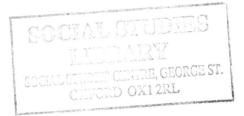

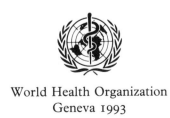

World Health Organization
Geneva 1993

WHO Library Cataloguing in Publication Data

The Urban health crisis : strategies for health for all in the face of rapid urbanization : report of the Technical Discussions at the Forty-fourth World Health Assembly.

1.Urban health 2.Urbanization 3.Health policy

ISBN 92 4 156159 9   (NLM Classification: WA 380)

The World Health Organization welcomes requests for permission to reproduce or translate its publications in part or in full. Applications and enquiries should be addressed to the Office of Publications, World Health Organization, Geneva, Switzerland, which will be glad to provide the latest information on any changes made to the text, plans for new editions, and reprints and translations already available.

© World Health Organization 1993

TYPESET IN INDIA
PRINTED IN ENGLAND

93/9628–Macmillan/Clays–7000

THE URBAN HEALTH CRISIS

Strategies for health for all in the face of rapid urbanization

Contents

Preface

The current rapid growth in urban areas is driven by the search for employment, changes in production and marketing practices, the direct and indirect effects of development policies, and the search for a better life. By the year 2000, most of the world's population will live in large towns or cities, and the urban setting will play a major part in determining their health status. This represents a daunting challenge, particularly to municipal governments, which must ensure that essential services, such as health care, water supply, housing, and solid waste management, can keep pace with the growing needs of their populations.

Recognizing the importance of this problem, the World Health Organization selected urban health as the subject of the Technical Discussions at the Forty-fourth World Health Assembly in 1991. The Discussions focused on ways of raising awareness and mobilizing the community to participate with local agencies and institutions in improving environmental and health conditions in urban areas. The participants concluded that municipal health planning must promote intersectoral action, involving local government agencies, community organizations, nongovernmental organizations, and the private sector. The report of the Discussions is now being published in the hope that this message, together with the other conclusions emanating from the Discussions, will reach a wider audience and stimulate local governments to implement a health-for-all policy at city level.

The World Health Organization is grateful to the many people who helped in the preparations for the Discussions, as well as to the participants themselves. The key role of Dr John Ashton, Department of Public Health, University of Liverpool, Liverpool, England, in acting as rapporteur for the Discussions and in writing this report, is particularly acknowledged.

Foreword

By the year 2000 a majority of the world's population will live in large towns or cities. For most city-dwellers the urban setting will play a major part in determining their level of health. Moreover, it is becoming increasingly clear that the way in which we choose to organize and run our cities will be critical to the future ecology of the planet itself. These essential facts lie behind the recent emergence of a sense of crisis about the condition of the world's cities, about urban health, and about the situation of the urban poor.

It is estimated that during the period 1990 to 2020, the total world population will increase from 5.2 thousand million to about 7.8 thousand million, i.e., by about 50%. During the same period, the urban population will double. In many countries the entire increase in population is taking place in urban areas. In the early stages of city development, migration tends to be the dominant influence on urban growth. Later, natural increase usually becomes the main reason for sustained growth. One effect of this growth is that the populations of some cities in developing countries are expected to become extremely large by the end of the century. These include Mexico City (32 million), São Paulo (26 million), Bombay, Calcutta, Jakarta and Rio de Janeiro (over 16 million each), Cairo, Manila and Seoul (12 million).

In many countries the urban population has outgrown the sustainable yield from surrounding land, forest, and water systems, with resulting environmental degradation, decreased agricultural production, so-called natural disasters, scarcity of water for drinking and sanitation, and increased landlessness. The result is poverty and ill health affecting both rural and urban populations, combined with severe ecological pressures on the environment.

Good health depends to a large extent on a good environment. In many cities there are large differences in health between different areas, principally because of inadequate housing and sanitation, which are in turn related to a lack of disposable income. To take a simple example, infant mortality may vary as much as fivefold between adjacent urban neighbourhoods. The urban crisis is probably having at least as great an impact on health as any one of the familiar captains in the army of death—malaria, tuberculosis, coronary heart disease, or cancer. Rapid migration to the towns often leads to a breakdown of families and social networks of support. This in turn has been a fundamental factor in the occurrence of two escalating pandemics—AIDS and drug abuse—and in the high prevalence of mental illness. The overwhelming of the urban infrastructure has also created the conditions under which microbes flourish. The dramatic upsurge of cholera is the latest, and perhaps not the last, example of this phenomenon.

The selection of urban health as the subject of the Technical Discussions at the Forty-fourth World Health Assembly was a highly significant turning-point and marked explicit recognition of the importance of this issue. In his opening remarks the Director-General of WHO, Dr H. Nakajima, reminded the audience that urbanization was not necessarily bad in itself. It became a problem when the rate of growth of the urban population exceeded the capacity of the infrastructure to absorb and support it. The context for the discussions was set by Dr Nakajima's statement to the Executive Board, in which he referred to the need for a new paradigm for health, which would take account of the changing demographic situation and the socioeconomic realities of the 1990s.

Such a paradigm must consist of a world view in which health is seen as an investment and as central both to economic development and to the quality of life. Health and the impact of proposed developments upon health must in future be essential elements of social and economic planning. The creation of a broad and sustainable infrastructure is also essential if health is to be improved.

As Chairman of the Technical Discussions, I referred to six imperatives which in my opinion were prerequisites for improved urban health. These were: to decentralize, putting the emphasis on action at the municipal level; to mobilize all agencies and everyone who can help in city networks; to invest in safe drinking-water and wastewater disposal; to help the poor increase their incomes and improve their dwellings; to provide families with a range of sustainable health services in or near their homes with the main emphasis on family planning; and finally to ask the poor, with humility, to identify their own needs.

One recurring theme in the Technical Discussions was environmental health. It is essential that there should be a balance between population size and distribution and the environmental infrastructure. The situation of new migrants living in illegal housing poses a particular challenge to city and government administrations and there is an urgent need to review policy as it affects such people. Recognition and legitimization of squatters are often needed before a sanitary infrastructure and the other basics of primary health care can be provided. Nor is a narrow sanitary view any longer adequate in tackling the environmental aspects of urban health. The ecological crisis has now led us to realize that urban development must take account not only of the direct impact of development on human health, but also of the wider and longer-term threat to health presented by neglect of the ecological impact of urban lifestyles. In environmental health, as in so many other aspects of urban health, there is a shortage of data on which to base policy. There is a need for a much more active approach to the dissemination of existing knowledge and to the provision of technical support for environmental health development and for innovation, particularly of a kind that can be carried out at low cost by neighbourhood action or by small-scale entrepreneurs.

A second theme in the Technical Discussions was the organization of urban health systems. The group felt that there was a need for an urgent reappraisal of urban health systems and for the sharing of experience between urban areas. The following factors were identified as being of particular importance in developing appropriate urban health systems:

- *Public awareness.* There is a need to make the public aware of the real issues involved and to obtain practical local data so that interventions can be targeted at the groups that need them most. There is a particular need for comparisons to be made of health indicators between different intracity areas because such comparisons can be used to develop a common agenda for local residents, professional health workers, and politicians.

- *Reorientation of services.* At present, referral hospitals are heavily used for first-contact care, and this inappropriate use of specialized facilities tends to divert resources from those at greatest risk. However, there was general support for the development of local reference health centres combining health promotion, preventive medicine, primary health care, and maternal and child health services and providing outpatient and day-surgery care. Examples may be cited of centres of this kind that are well integrated into the health system and enjoy high levels of public support. They can provide a powerful focus for community development.

- *Leadership, organization, and management.* There was considerable emphasis on the need to decentralize responsibility and authority for running urban health systems both to the city level from the central government and to the neighbourhood level within cities. This calls for a new kind of political and professional leadership that accepts a facilitating rather than a controlling role. There is also an urgent need for training in the management skills required to implement such an approach effectively.

- *Urban capacity-building.* The magnitude of the tasks facing city government is often frightening, and some of the city administrations with the worst combination of issues to be tackled are also the most fragile. This poses a challenge to the way in which many health workers regard the public as passive consumers of care rather than as coproducers and maintainers of health. The implications for institutions training health workers are considerable, notably as regards the orientation both of training and of research.

The World Health Organization (WHO) and other international bodies have an important role in the organization of urban health systems. International agencies must in future include an assessment of the impact on health, as well as on the environment, in all their planning processes. Health issues and health agencies and departments are at present often left out of the relevant discussions. Health considerations must be pressed wherever decisions about social and economic policy are made. WHO can assist urban development in developing countries by promoting methodologies, research, documentation, institution-building, and training, and providing opportunities for the exchange of ideas and of true stories of both mistakes and achievements. WHO can also take a leading role in stimulating the collaboration of other international agencies and ensuring that the impact of development strategies on health is made explicit. It can also continue to provide progressive leadership by ensuring that it is setting a good example in the way it conducts its affairs—in particular, by the adoption of a more proactive advocacy role on behalf of the urban poor.

A third theme in the Technical Discussions was that of city networks for health. The sharing of experience in the implementation of health-for-all strategies at the local level is an important and effective way of strengthening city action. There are now a number of examples of international networks of collaborating cities including Metropolis, CITYNET, and WHO's Healthy Cities Project in the European Region. Since 1986, this project has enjoyed a high level of success in encouraging cities in Europe and elsewhere to form networks for sharing experience in the area of health promotion. This approach should be encouraged on a global scale as one way of tackling the urban health crisis.

A fourth theme was that of urban policies and health status. It seems that today, as in the past, the city may be an appropriate level at which to focus on developments in public health. In nineteenth-century Europe and North America it was the cities that, when confronted by the epidemic diseases that ravaged undernourished populations living in squalid housing, responded to the challenge. Many of the factors that have a major impact on health are subject to rules, regulations, and laws that depend on urban policies. Housing, water supply, air and water pollution, food supply, the control of pests and disease vectors, and the development of local transport systems are typical examples of services for which sound urban policies must be adopted and applied. There is an urgent need to strengthen local government so that it is in a position to play its part in improving urban health as effectively as posssible. Health education and health promotion also have an important role in setting the agenda and raising awareness so that local models of good practice can be developed. Finally, health can only be achieved within cities if there is a real and vital partnership between the relevant agencies and the city-dwellers themselves, and much more effective collaboration between all agencies and interests with a role in urban development. These are the areas on which we must now concentrate.

Sir Donald Acheson
*General Chairman, Technical
Discussions, Fourty-fourth World
Health Assembly*

Resolution WHA 44.27

adopted by the Forty-fourth World Health Assembly, May 1991

The Forty-fourth World Health Assembly,

Noting that between 1950 and 1990 the world's urban population rose from 734 million to 2390 million (more than triple), or from 29% to 45% of the total population, and that the increase is continuing;

Aware that most of the increase was in cities of developing countries, whose urban population increased five-fold, from 286 million in 1950 to 1515 million in 1990;

Noting that annual urban population growth rates of 3% or more have been common in developing countries, and may continue over the next 20 years; that such growth exceeds the capacity of a city to provide adequate resources, housing, employment, and services, and results in the exposure of increasing numbers of urban dwellers to the hazards of poverty, unemployment, inadequate housing, poor sanitation, pollution, disease vectors, poor transport, and psychological and social stress;

Taking account of the conclusions and recommendations of the Technical Discussions held during the Forty-fourth World Health Assembly;

Recalling action taken by WHO for health development in urban areas;

Recognizing the need for the reappraisal of urban health systems so that they contribute to the promotion of urban health in the context of health for all;

Noting that the WHO Commission on Health and Environment considers urbanization a major driving force of development;

Aware of the attention to urban development in the programmes of the United Nations Centre for Human Settlements, UNDP and UNEP, and in the preparations for the United Nations Conference on Environment and Development in 1992;

1. URGES Member States:

    (1) to prevent excessive urban population growth by:
        (a) developing national policies that maintain urban population in balance with infrastructure and services, and that give due attention to family planning;
        (b) adjusting urban and rural development policies to provide incentives for the public, industry, the

private sector and government agencies to prevent excessive concentration of population in potential urban problem areas;

(2) to strengthen the capacity for healthy urban development by:

    (a) adjusting and implementing policies at all levels to render urban development sustainable and to preserve an environment supportive of health;

    (b) assessing the impact on health of the policies of agencies concerned with energy, food, agriculture, macroeconomic planning, housing, industry, transport and communications, education and social welfare, and adjusting them better to promote healthy communities and a healthy environment in cities;

    (c) developing suitable structures and processes for coherent intersectoral and community participation in the planning and implementation of urban development policies;

(3) to ensure that responsibilities for urban development and management, including health and social services, are decentralized from the national level to a level compatible with efficient and integrated management and technological requirements;

(4) to give priority to the development, reorientation, and strengthening of urban health services based on the primary health care approach, including appropriate referral services, with particular emphasis on response to the needs of the urban poor;

(5) to strengthen effective and full community participation in urban development by promoting strong partnerships between government and community organizations, including nongovernmental organizations, the private sector, and the local people;

(6) to develop national and international networks of cities and communities for health in order to increase community participation and gain political support for technical programmes to improve health services and environmental health;

(7) to improve information and research in order to relate health data to environmental conditions and health services; and to measure health differentials between parts of towns or cities in order to guide municipal authorities in the planning and management of health development programmes;

2. CALLS ON international agencies:

   (1) to give proper attention in their programmes to the relation between the urban crisis and the growing degradation of the global environment;
   (2) to consider environmental, social, and health needs when deciding on their priorities and allocations, and take into account the impact of those decisions on health;
   (3) to develop new ways of providing national governments, municipal authorities, and community organizations with support in order to help them tackle urban health problems as part of urban development;

3. REQUESTS the Director-General:

   (1) to further strengthen WHO's information base and ensure the availability of data to countries and cities so that they may deal with the human and environmental health aspects of urban development;
   (2) to strengthen technical cooperation in health development in urban areas with and between Member States in order to increase awareness of the needs of the urban poor, develop national skills in meeting these needs, and support the extension of city networks for health throughout the world;
   (3) to promote regional networks and interdisciplinary panels of experts and community leaders to advise on health aspects of urban development;
   (4) to submit a report on progress in the implementation of this resolution to a future World Health Assembly through the Executive Board.

Introduction

The selection of urban health as the subject of the Technical Discussions at the Forty-fourth World Health Assembly was a highly significant turning-point. It marked the explicit recognition by the World Health Organization of the impending health crisis in urban areas, and indicated a distinct shift of emphasis in public health thinking. Previously, there had been an almost exclusive preoccupation with the problems of health in rural areas; however, it was becoming clear that, although there were some issues that were specific to either the rural or the urban situation, the core issues of the balance between population and resources, the movement of people, and the process of rapid urbanization had implications for health and well-being in both rural and urban areas. The resulting problems of both rural and urban areas are interrelated and indivisible.

The recent emergence of concern about urban health can be easily explained from a review of the growth and distribution of the world population. The number of people living in towns and cities throughout the world is growing rapidly, and by the end of the century the number of urban dwellers will exceed the number of rural dwellers for the first time in human history. The large-scale movement of people to the towns, which began in Europe with industrialization, has become a global phenomenon. The urbanization process may be seen as one that begins with movement from country villages to small and medium-sized towns, which rapidly become big cities, and that progresses to intercountry migration and the movement of people from the poorer to the richer parts of the world.

Rapid urbanization is now most marked in developing countries, where urban growth rates of 3% or more each year are not uncommon. Such growth rates, which lead to a doubling of population every twenty years, are so high that the local authorities are unable to keep pace with the demand for basic services such as housing, water, and sanitation.

This rapid urban growth is a result of two factors: the movement of rural populations into towns on the one hand, and the natural increase resulting from a surplus of births over deaths in urban populations, on the other. In general, as countries reach higher levels of urbanization, the impact of migration becomes less important and that of natural increase more important, especially among low-income groups.

The problems observed in cities 150 years ago are all to be found today, on a much bigger scale and with much worse consequences. However, some things are different; science has provided some remarkably effective tools, such as immunization and family planning methods which, if made available to populations and properly used, can help prevent a vast amount of human misery, ill health, and loss of life. Many cities have well-developed public services and health systems which, if properly managed, can make a significant contribution to this process. Unfortunately, these services and systems are frequently bureaucratic, compartmentalized, and ineffective. They fail to connect with other organizations that have a contribution to make, and alienate the people they are supposed to serve. Sometimes it may seem that public organizations are run more for the benefit of the employees than for the public.

In many countries, urban populations are now so large that they have outgrown the capacity of the surrounding agricultural areas to provide the food and raw materials needed to sustain them, and they overload the natural water systems with human and industrial waste. As a result there is a vicious circle of environmental deterioration, reduced agricultural production, "natural disasters", and increased pauperization and landlessness. In addition, the idea that the cities offer a better life than the depressed countryside is encouraging migration to the cities just when decreased agricultural production is reducing the availability of food and increasing its price.

As a result there is poverty and ill health in both rural and urban populations, together with severe ecological pressures on the environment. About half the inhabitants of cities in the developing world are likely to be living in conditions of extreme poverty and, until this basic problem is tackled, the total number of premature deaths in developing cities will continue to increase. One difficulty in taking effective action to deal with the situation is the lack of even basic information on birth and death rates, the incidence of disease, and environmental conditions. When such information is available it is usually found that, in urban areas, the health of the poor is much worse than that of the better-off and that, contrary to popular belief, it is no better and may be much worse than that of people living in rural areas.

2

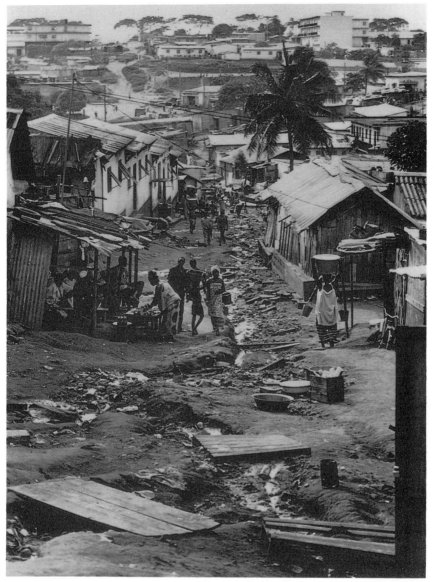

WHO/UN/B. Wolff (20952)

Crowded, makeshift housing and inadequate water and sanitation are associated with increased mortality and morbidity due to communicable diseases, especially gastrointestinal and respiratory diseases.

Nor are the problems of the urban poor confined to the developing countries. In the industrialized parts of the world, cities are to be found at many different stages of development. In some places, new cities are still being established, and old ones continue to grow and to be remodelled. In others, once-great cities are undergoing a rapid decline, with increasing pollution, deteriorating physical infrastructure, and inner-city decay, as well as the loss of young and skilled people to economically more rewarding areas. The populations left behind tend to have a high proportion of old and sick people, with more social stress and weaker networks of social support. All of this is made worse by the limited access to health and social services that is the usual lot of the poor.

The health consequences of poverty in the cities of the developed world include a high incidence of heart disease and stroke, cancer, drug and alcohol abuse, accidents, violence, and sexually transmitted diseases, including HIV infection and AIDS. In the cities of the developing world, a high incidence of these conditions exists alongside traditional health problems such as high maternal, perinatal, infant, and child death rates and infections and parasitic diseases that have thrived under squalid urban conditions.

The trends of growth and decay in cities have been accompanied by dramatic changes in traditional social structures—the decline of the three-generation family and the changing expectations of women and of marriage, together with many changes in personal and social expectations and goals. Accompanying these changes have been increasingly mixed societies with multiracial and multicultural communities becoming commonplace.

The widespread breakdown of family structures and networks of social support has been an important factor in such escalating threats to world health as AIDS and drug abuse and the high incidence of mental illness. The dramatic increases in population are in many parts of the world accompanied by considerable increases in the proportion of people who live to an old age; this in itself is creating a crisis of social and medical care throughout the world in both rural and urban areas.

All these aspects of the urban condition have combined to throw the spotlight on the urban health crisis and to challenge governments, nongovernmental organizations, local health systems, and ordinary citizens to do something now before the situation is completely out of control.

Chapter 1

Health and the cities: a global overview

Trends in urbanization

Urban growth is fuelled by poverty, the search for work, insecurity of land tenure, changes in farming and in industrial processes, and the growth of service industries. Policies for economic development that tend to lead to concentration of opportunities for work and of pools of skilled labour in towns and cities are accompanied by a widespread view that cities offer a better life than the increasingly depressed rural areas. Despite prophecies that the cities are doomed, they remain in the front line of innovation and change and, for many, offer dreams of an urban Utopia; millions of young people around the world still flock into cities.

Slum conditions are to be found in all the cities of developing countries. However, the extent of these conditions and of actual homelessness varies from city to city. In some cities, such as Calcutta and Bombay, a majority of the population lives in slums. However, in addition to the large numbers of slum-dwellers there are also many people who are completely homeless and who live on the streets. This is a particular problem in, for example, Calcutta, Manila, and even in Los Angeles, where as many as 50 000 people may be homeless.

Meanwhile urbanization contributes to changes in local ecosystems and the biosphere that affect the health and living conditions of both urban and rural populations. These changes have produced a burden of ill health and disability that is of crisis proportions in some Third World cities, especially in countries that have stagnant economies and heavy burdens of external debt to banks and institutions in the developed world. This crisis is deepened when health service resources are used inequitably or are misused on low-priority or inappropriate programmes.

5

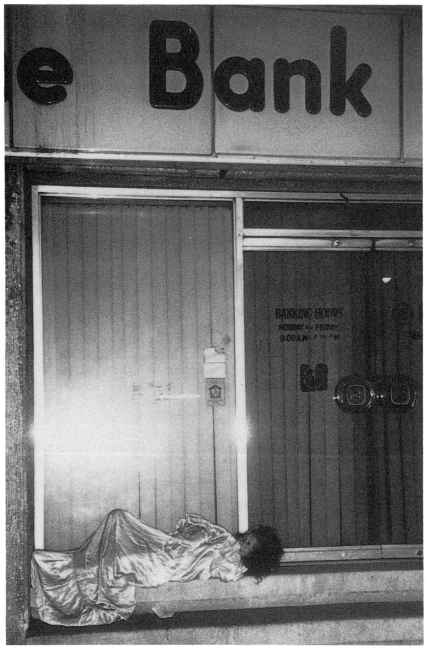

WHO/Zafar (20917)

The bank houses the wealth of the few; its entrance offers a place to sleep for one of the many "street children".

- Urban populations have greatly increased in the past 40 years.

- The greatest increase has been in developing countries.

- Urban populations will increase even more rapidly in the next 35 years with an explosive growth of cities in developing countries.

- Although the number of rural dwellers will increase, their share of the total population will not: people living in cities will become a majority of the world population, and the proportion of people in developing countries living in cities will approach that of the developed world.

Factors that have an impact on health include:

- Rapid and massive urban population growth, both in an increasing number of "megacities" and in smaller cities.

- Large populations in squatter settlements and shanty towns often occupying urban land subject to landslides, floods, and other natural hazards.

- Increased population density, overcrowding, congestion, and traffic, and the spread of unsuitable residential patterns.

- Ever-growing numbers of people living in extreme poverty, many of them—especially women and children—at high social risk.

- Increasing biological, chemical, and physical pollution of air, water, and land from industrialization, transportation, energy production, and commercial and domestic wastes.

- Financial and administrative inability to provide a sanitary infrastructure, promote adequate employment and housing, manage wastes, and ensure security, environmental controls, and health and social services.

Quality of life

Productivity and poverty are two indicators that are useful in assessing the quality of life of urban dwellers. Productivity is a measure of the efficiency of large cities as engines of economic development and producers of amenities. A minority of the population of developing countries living in cities produces the majority of the gross domestic product (GDP). The extreme cases include Bangkok, where 10% of the national population produces 80% of Thailand's GDP, and Dhaka, which contains 4% of Bangladesh's population and 60% of its manufacturing establishments. Among the reasons for urban productivity are the economies of scale and the benefits that come from a variety of productive facilities being close to each other and to a large market for their products, and the tendency of cities to attract the better educated, the skilled, and those with disposable income. These factors make it feasible to provide an efficient infrastructure and services, including medical care services. However, the possibility of doing so may be reduced because of a lack of investment, wasted resources, poor management, and inadequate political and social organization.

Both developed and developing countries have examples of places where poorly managed urban development, together with economic stagnation, has led to reduced production, higher prices

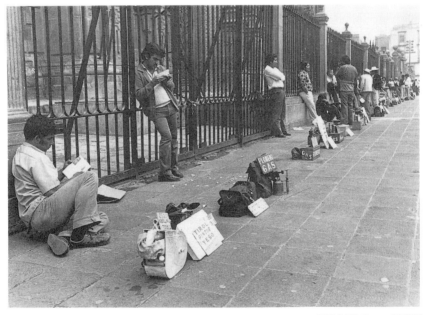

WHO/ILO/D. Bregnard (20951)

Job-seekers in urban areas are increasing faster than municipal economies. Is this employment? Repairmen offering their services by the roadside, Mexico City.

and unemployment levels, cuts in public expenditure for social services, higher borrowing rates, and a decline in infrastructure investment. Urbanization may either help or hinder rural development. The rural economy may be supported through increased demand for products and through people who have moved to the towns sending cash to their families. On the other hand, urban consumption may place excessive demands on the hinterland's resources, as well as causing damage through the disposal of waste. Although comprehensive statistics on urban poverty are lacking and the ways in which it is measured differ, it is likely that about a quarter of the world's population—1100 million people—are living in poverty, most of them in developing countries, and that about one-third of urban dwellers in developing countries live in substandard housing or are homeless.

Health risks are increased by poverty because basic needs go unmet and the poor are exposed to additional hazards. In most industrialized countries the urban poor are a small but growing minority. They suffer the effects of deprivation and are increasingly afflicted by the evils associated with industrialization: toxic pollution, congestion, noise, heart disease, mental illness, drug abuse, crime, and violence. In developing countries, poor and near-poor populations are much larger, economic conditions worse, infrastructures undeveloped, personal safety more threatened, goods scarcer, and illiteracy more widespread. Most social development policies have tried to counter the effects of poverty but the interventions have usually helped relatively few people. Rarely do policies attack the root causes of poverty—the need for land reform, low pay and inequitable wage structures, insecure housing tenure, poor protection for workers, social isolation, and poor health. Meanwhile, the potential contribution to improved well-being of those working in the informal economy has seldom been fully realized, although they make major contributions to house-building, the recycling of waste, and the production of cheap goods and services essential to urban enterprise and to consumers.

Urban growth and community organization

Newcomers to growing towns and cities have always been likely to find themselves living in the most adverse surroundings. Some 140 years ago, 300 000 refugees from the Irish potato famine landed in Liverpool, England. Between 60 000 and 80 000 of them settled in the city at a time when the resident population was 120 000, living predominantly in the poorest parts of the city, where they recreated as best they could a village and parish structure within the town. The inevitable result of this influx of desperately poor and starving people, forced to live in crowded and insanitary slum conditions, was a massive outbreak of typhus, accompanied by epidemics of smallpox, measles, scarlet fever, tuberculosis and, in 1849, cholera.

This type of experience is being echoed today around the world, often on a much greater scale than in Liverpool in 1848. Not only are there countless disadvantaged high-risk groups living in unhealthy conditions, but the situation is further grossly compounded by serious socioeconomic problems and the crisis of international debt, which diverts financial resources from being used to further social justice among the urban poor. The groups that are most at risk in these circumstances are the illiterate, the unemployed, the homeless, the sick, and people who are stigmatized because of their lifestyles or alienated because they are refugees. Their unfavourable situation is compounded by their limited access to good primary health care.

Squatting in shanty dwellings in the least desirable areas, often on the edge of town, perhaps in an area of swamp or stagnant water, without sanitary infrastructure, vulnerable to natural disaster, flood, and infection, millions of people struggle to survive. Often the efforts made by communities to organize and house themselves, or to provide themselves with services, are actively opposed by government authorities or professional groups who feel their own position to be in some way threatened. Shanty towns may be cleared and people compulsorily removed from areas where they have invested their limited funds and their labour in trying to create the beginnings of a community, while their contributions to greater well-being through the informal economy often go unrecognized. Poor city-dwellers often have to pay high amounts to private vendors for limited water supplies, while the public services that are provided are often imposed in a paternalistic and patronizing manner which fails to recognize the knowledge and skills of the local people. Public services throughout the world usually have a centralized and compartmentalized character, which removes them from the people they are supposed to serve, at the same time failing to capitalize on the advantages of providing services in a horizontal and integrated, rather than in a vertical and specialized, manner.

The impact of urbanization on health

Physical, economic, social, and cultural aspects of city life all have an important influence on health. They exert their effect through such processes as population movement, industrialization, and changes in the architectural and physical environment and in social organization. Health is also affected in particular cities by climate, terrain, population density, housing stock, the nature of economic activity, income distribution, transport systems, and opportunities for leisure and recreation. The impact on health is not the simple total of all these factors, but the effect of their synergistic action, the whole being greater than the sum of the parts.

In Europe and North America, three overlapping phases of public health can be identified from the mid-nineteenth to the late twentieth century. The first phase began in the industrialized cities in response to the appalling toll of death and disease among the urban poor living in abject squalor. The displacement of large numbers of people from the land by their landlords, who wished to take advantage of the increased productivity obtained by applying scientific agricultural procedures, enhanced the attraction of the growing cities which appeared to offer country people opportunities for self-improvement. The results were massive population movements, disruption of the prevailing pattern of rural life, and the rapid creation of large slum areas.

The organized response of local and national governments included the introduction of legislation and the use of specially trained medical and environmental health officers to address the predominantly environmental threats to health with considerable effect. The focus of this movement was on improving standards of housing and sanitation and providing bacteriologically safe water and food. This initial public health movement with its emphasis on environmental change was, in time, eclipsed by one based rather on personal preventive action, made possible by advances in bacteriology, immunology, and the promotion of mechanical methods of birth control. This preventive phase was in turn superseded by the therapeutic era, starting in the 1930s with the advent of insulin and the sulfonamide drugs, to be followed later by antibiotics and a great number of scientifically based treatments. The beginning of this period coincided with the apparent conquest of the infectious diseases in developed countries, on the one hand, and an increased involvement of governments in direct patient care through insurance-based and public health care systems, on the other. Historically it marked the weakening of public health departments, and of the role of general medical practitioners and a shift of power and resources to hospital-based services that lasted until well into the 1970s.

Since the early 1970s a comprehensive approach to health development has emerged, combining environmental change with appropriate preventive and therapeutic interventions, especially for high-risk groups such as children, mothers, the elderly, and the disabled. The origins of this so-called "new public health" can be traced to a growing awareness of the limitations of therapy and a greater understanding of the reasons for health improvements in the past. Ideas about health have been changing: the traditional "sanitary" view, focusing on the environment, and the more recent mechanical, biomedical view, focusing on the human body, have been superseded by more holistic concepts which recognize that health is fundamentally an ecological matter and must deal with the linked phenomena of population growth, urbanization, consumption, environmental degradation, premature death and disability, and poor services. There is a growing awareness of the need to take a horizontal rather than a vertical view of public health as "the science and art of preventing disease, prolonging life and promoting health through the organized efforts of society" (*1*).

Unless such an integrative view is taken, health service interventions can have only a limited impact on the health of populations. Children whose lives are saved by immunization may nevertheless die from malnutrition, while sanitary improvements alone will have little or no effect on many infectious diseases. Public water systems may be constructed, but the effective delivery of safe water to slum populations needs well-organized and well-managed water companies and the ability to maintain plant and equipment. The reduction of respiratory disease that is due in part to air pollution depends on controlling traffic and exhaust emissions, the location of industrial premises, the nature of industrial processes, and the types of facility used for domestic heating and cooking—in short, it needs an intersectoral approach.

In theory, a city's compactness and high productivity can support the promotion and protection of health, but, while such threats to health as air pollution may affect all social groups, it is the growing numbers of urban poor in all countries who are exposed to the most health-threatening elements in the urban environment. Health needs are greatest in Third World cities whose health problems include both the infectious diseases and malnutrition traditionally associated with developing countries and the non-infectious diseases associated with development (heart disease, stroke, cancer, accidents, suicide, alcohol dependence, other drug-related problems, and mental disorders). In addition, the new scourge of AIDS, which appears to be a particularly acute urban problem, is a significant threat to public health in both the developing and the developed world. Populations that are geographically concentrated are potentially capable of improving their health by using technical and social resources to alter the physical environment and improve living and working conditions. Whether they will actually do so depends on the strength of their social networks, the nature of their social practices, and the extent of their commitment to social justice.

Poor health is most frequent among the so-called marginal or underclass populations, which are increasing in many cities in both the developing and the developed world. These are people who are classed as minorities, whose poverty is reinforced because they work for low rates of pay in the informal economy, who lack social organization, and who often have no legal status as citizens. Adequate nutrition, hygiene, and housing are likely to be beyond their grasp and they may be exploited when they try to meet their basic needs; for example, poor slum-dwellers may have to pay more for limited amounts of water, often unsafe, from private sources than the better-off pay for piped supplies. Unemployment and many types of insecurity affect their resistance to disease. Frequently they have no access to the health and social services, even emergency services.

Health is also affected when people are not educated to a level permitting them to improve their income and living conditions, to eat properly, and to protect themselves and their families from the many threats to their health.

Economic factors

During the past 10 years, most developing countries have experienced a stagnation of economic growth and development. Many have heavy external debts so that a major part of the national income has to go to meet interest payments. Frequently the result has been a decline in per capita income and a rise in real prices. This has reduced the resources available for investment in the development and maintenance of the urban infrastructure and public sector services. These conditions have led to the deterioration of urban environments and the reduction of public services with negative effects on the health, quality of life, and productivity of all city dwellers, but especially the poor.

The social and health consequences of economic conditions in general have been aggravated by:

- uncontrolled industrialization and exploitation of natural resources, causing pollution, higher prices, a decline in real incomes, unemployment, reduced public spending, and ecologically unsound development;

- rates of population growth from migration and natural increase that exceed the ability of social and economic development to keep pace with them;

- the exclusion of many slum-dwellers from full civic and economic status, thus creating an underclass which survives within the informal economy with little security of land, housing, employment, or education.

Urban health problems

In rapidly urbanizing areas, the lack of even basic statistics about life, death, disease, and access to public services makes it difficult to describe with any accuracy the effects of life in such areas on health. The available information may appear to show that health levels in the cities are better than those in the rural villages. However, when urban statistics are specially collected and analysed in ways that make comparisons possible within cities, huge differences are usually found. The health consequences of urban poverty in the cities of developed countries include a high incidence of heart disease, stroke, cancer, drug and alcohol abuse, accidents, violence, AIDS, and sexually transmitted disease. In cities in the developing world these conditions now exist side by side with traditional health problems such as high maternal, perinatal, infant, and child mortality. The urban areas of the developing countries are thus getting the worst of both worlds.

Although the full extent of urban health problems and their relative frequency among different groups of city-dwellers, are not known, studies have clearly shown that the odds against children surviving to adult life and against people living to old age are greater for those city-dwellers who are faced with malnutrition, inadequate shelter, poor sanitation, pollution, poor public transport, and psychological and social stress due to economic deprivation. The lack of proper information hides the extent of the unmet needs and makes it difficult to plan for the most effective and efficient use of limited resources.

Communicable diseases

Communicable diseases flourish where resistance levels are low, immunization is inadequate, and the environmental barriers against their spread are weak; poor nutrition makes people, particularly the young and feeble, more vulnerable to infection. The situation is made worse by overcrowding, by the exposure of populations to diseases to which they have never been exposed before, and by the multiplication of animal and insect hosts because of environmental, behavioural and ecological changes.

Environmental conditions favouring the spread of communicable diseases include insufficient and unsafe water supplies, poor sanitation, inadequate disposal of solid wastes, inadequate drainage of surface water, poor personal and domestic hygiene, inadequate housing, and overcrowding. Many of these are due to a lack of facilities and services but human behaviour, often culturally based, may be an important factor. For example, new migrants may persist in unhygienic traditional practices, such as using surface water, or dealing with faeces in ways that are unsuited to towns and cities.

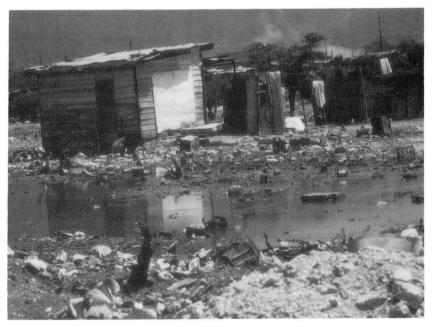

Standing water due to poor drainage leads to a steady toll of faecal-oral diseases, urban schistosomiasis, and mosquito-borne infections such as malaria and dengue fever.

HIV infection and AIDS have come to be seen as a major threat to health within a very few years, and there is a concentration of cases in urban areas. Poverty, coexisting general infection, unsafe sexual behaviour, intravenous drug abuse, and use of unsafe blood and blood products are all contributory factors to a problem that needs to be tackled energetically, creatively, and on a broad front. Effective intervention requires the cooperation of many agencies from the public, private, and voluntary sectors and raises challenging questions about cultural and religious beliefs and practices. Faced with such problems as HIV infection and AIDS, the public health services have a duty to the population as a whole to be practical, pragmatic, and persistent.

Noncommunicable diseases

Much of the burden of chronic disease and trauma, including poisoning, burns, and injuries, is associated with urban environments and lifestyles, inadequate early detection and treatment of disease, and poor health education.

Structural defects in housing, inadequate means of transport, and poorly organized workplaces contribute to the burden of noncommunicable disease by creating unsafe environments. Sources of risk include indoor air pollution, inadequate provisions for escape in the event of fire or explosion, road traffic hazards, poorly constructed workplaces, and unsafe building materials.

The siting of human settlements in relation to areas used for industrial and domestic waste disposal is crucial in protecting people against pollution of the air, water, and soil. Squatters and slum-dwellers are particularly at risk, because they often have no alternative but to live in close proximity to dirty industries, contaminated water courses, or swamps, and in areas that are subject to landslip, flooding, and other "natural" hazards. Exposure to toxic and caustic substances is growing with the increased use of chemicals in industry and in the home. Chemical contamination of food, water, and air can have chronic effects, some of which are probably still not known. Accidents in the course of the manufacture, storage, and transport of goods can be a particular problem in built-up areas. Air pollution has many adverse effects on health. The toxic and degenerative effects of lead from vehicle emissions are now well documented. Various emissions and dusts contribute to the occurrence of smog and acid rain with harmful effects on plants, animals, and humans. In developing countries, domestic pollution caused by inadequately ventilated cooking and heating devices puts hundreds of millions of people at risk.

Mental disorder

Urban life can give people greater opportunities to develop their own interests and activities since, with so many people concentrated in a limited geographical area, there is likely to be sufficient support for specialized facilities of various kinds. However, urban life has the drawback that it can increase the isolation of individuals and families. Social and emotional stress is likely to be severe among people new to city life and those without a secure home and livelihood. Urban stress often manifests itself in depression, anxiety, suicide, alcohol and drug abuse, crime, and family violence. Increases in mental disorder among older city-dwellers have been reported, as well as increases in such problems as juvenile delinquency, teenage pregnancy, and violence.

Emotional disturbance is not uncommon in children who have moved from the country to the city, and city children living in slums or on the streets are often open to exploitation; drug addiction, crime, prostitution, and suicide are all fates that threaten children living on the margins of slum society. Studies of new migrants have

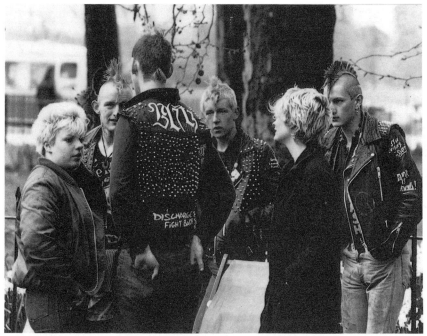

WHO/ILO/J. Maillard (20935)

Young people in cities may have increased opportunities for personal development, but are also vulnerable to problems such as juvenile delinquency, demoralization and despair, alienation, drug abuse, and suicide.

shown an association between physical and mental ill health and poverty and insecurity. Related problems include exposure to noise, frequent household moves, segregation and discrimination, lack of privacy, and a high risk of being a victim of crime.

Vulnerable groups

The largest group at risk in the city is the urban poor. Poverty intensifies the risks that go with childhood, old age, being female, racial minority status, disability, and occupation. The poor are usually further afflicted by limited access to health, education, social, and other public services.

While all children in cities are vulnerable, poor children are especially so. Children who have no legal status or who are separated from their families are at the highest risk. It has been estimated that there are over 20 million homeless "street children" in Latin America alone. Although, on the whole, infant mortality in developing countries has been reduced, the rates remain high in poor urban communities. Despite successes in tackling the immunizable dis-

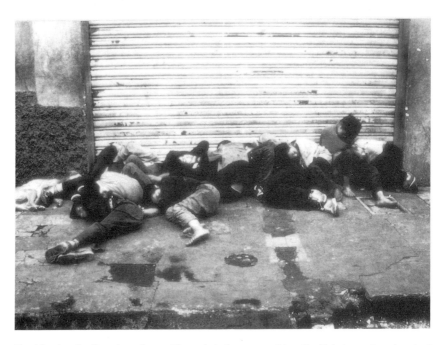

Rapid urbanization, together with social change and family disintegration, has led to the phenomenon of "street children", who are exposed to many serious health risks.

18

eases, each year 2.8 million children die from them and a further 3 million suffer chronic ill health as a result of them. One-third of children in developing countries weigh less than 2.5 kg at birth, and almost half the children in Africa show some signs of malnutrition. In some societies child labour is common and the exploitation and abandonment of children are condoned. Child abuse, a significant problem in many countries throughout the world, is concentrated in cities, and parental negligence contributes to injuries and poisoning by drugs and other chemicals.

Older children and adolescents are especially prone to death and injury from accidents and violence, and from drug and alcohol abuse. Some cities also report high rates of depression, suicide, and other manifestations of psychological stress among adolescents.

Women's health is undermined by poverty, poor education, and disadvantage and discrimination in the workplace. Women may be at a disadvantage from birth onwards because of inadequate nutrition, lack of education, heavy workloads, early marriage, and early and frequent pregnancies; their vulnerability increases when

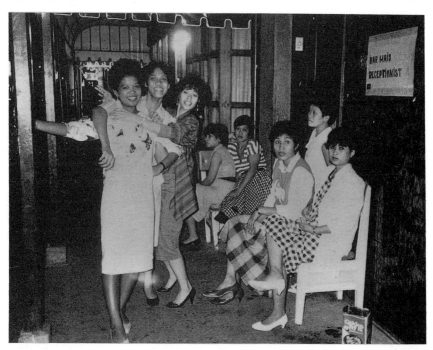

WHO/Zafar (20955)

In almost every city, there is a flourishing sex industry. The increasing AIDS problem—which affects not only the workers and their clients but the entire community—is focusing the attention of public health authorities on how to make this industry safer.

they have no partner. Inadequate contraception, unsafe abortion, lack of sanitation, and inferior health care explain why the risk of dying in childbirth is over 100 times greater among poor women from developing countries than among women from the industrialized countries. Prostitution, involving girls and boys as well as women, has grown to immense proportions in some developing countries; with the spread of AIDS, this has become an even more urgent public health issue. Women make an essential contribution to economic output in all countries, and their health is an important part of the world's human capital. Yet, throughout the world, women's health is compromised by low income, irregular work, and poor social and physical security.

The health needs of the elderly are increasing rapidly in all countries, along with their numbers. Increases in life expectancy have been most dramatic in developing countries during the past 50 years; projections indicate that, of the 1200 million people over 60 years of age expected to be alive in 2025, 71% will be in developing countries. These increases have economic and political implications, affecting social insurance and the provision of shelter, health care, and social support. The physical and mental health problems of aging are increased by poverty, vulnerability to crime, and the stress of adjusting one's lifestyle and coming to terms with loss of status, of income, and of friends and relatives. The culture of cities is often at odds with traditional practices of respect for one's elders.

The number of people with disabilities in the world has been estimated at 500 million and is projected to double by the early part of the next century. Four out of every five disabled people live in developing countries, and one-third of them are children. Relatively few countries are able to provide meaningful assistance, support, rehabilitation, and protection, leaving many to cope as best they can on the streets where they are subject to exploitation and chronic ill health. Disabled "street people", a large proportion of whom suffer from mental illness, are a significant problem in urban areas throughout the world, including some of the richest countries.

The number of people working in the informal economy in Third World cities is increasing faster than the number with stable incomes. Lacking regular jobs, these people are not covered by social insurance schemes, are often without protection against unsafe working conditions, and have limited access to health care.

Statistics on occupational health and accidents are poor in most developing countries, but it is generally thought that the accident rates in the informal sector of the economy are high. Workers and their families who live close to factories are often directly exposed to high levels of pollution and the effects of industrial accidents.

Chapter 2

Demographic factors

The increasing proportion of people living in cities and towns is now one of the main features of world development. From 1950 to 1985 the world's urban population almost trebled from 701 million to 1983 million, or from 25% to 41% of the total population. Population growth in the industrialized countries slowed over this period, so that most of the increase was in the cities of developing countries, where the urban population almost quadrupled from 286 million in 1950 to 1114 million in 1985. Overall, by the year 2000 51% of the world's 6300 million people are expected to be living in urban areas.

The urban population of developing countries is already larger than the combined urban populations of Europe, North America, and Japan. Overall, about 46% of urban dwellers live in cities with populations of at least 500 000. In general, population growth in large cities is much faster than overall population growth, so that urban problems in the future will be much greater even than they are already.

Urban growth rates in cities of developing countries have generally been 2–3 times those recorded in industrialized countries in the past, and continued annual increases of over 3% during the next 40 years have been forecast. The higher rates are mainly due to natural increase (excess of births over deaths) and migration, a further factor being the reclassification of urban areas. In the earlier stages of development, migration to cities is usually the most important cause of urban population growth, while later it is natural increase that dominates. In many developing countries a decline in urban fertility rates was anticipated as a result of increased literacy, improvements in income and employment, and the improved status of women, but this has not yet occurred to any significant degree.

As important factors in urban population growth, migration and natural increase are closely related. The relatively young age of new migrants to cities contributes to the high fertility rates and the low crude death rates. There is also a time lag of a generation between arrival in cities and the adoption of birth control practices. Fertility rates for migrants to cities tend to be high for some decades before their attitudes and behaviour change, especially when access to family planning information and services is limited.

The spectacular growth of the megacities has received increasing attention in recent years. In 1950, there was only one Third World city with a population of more than 5 million. In 1970, there were 11 and there are expected to be 35 by the year 2000; of these, 11 are predicted to have a population of 20–30 million. Even if these expectations are not realized, cities approaching this size present a considerable challenge to everybody; they are difficult to administer and manage, and there comes a point at which the benefits of population concentration and economy of scale are swamped by sheer numerical pressures on the infrastructure. However, the inhabitants of smaller cities make up the greater part of the world's urban population.

While the statistics for urban population growth are useful in describing the overall situation, each city is unique. To ensure good decisions and effective policies at the local level, each city must be assessed according to its specific characteristics, including its history, geography, culture, the natural resources of its hinterland, and its social, economic, and administrative capacity.

Statistics show that urban dwellers in developing countries have higher incomes, obtain a better education, and have better access to social and medical services than people living in rural areas. They also have better health status, as comparisons between the statistics for city populations and those for rural populations demonstrate. However, average figures often conceal extremely high morbidity and mortality rates for the urban poor, notably the slum-dwellers and the homeless, who may not appear in the statistics.

In developing countries, slum and squatter communities make up anything from one-third to a half, or more, of a city's population. Their members live in overcrowded conditions, lack sanitation and potable water, and have no secure employment. Slum communities are frequently illegal, exposed to floods and pollution, and beset with criminality and other serious social problems. Statistical averages generally mask their poor health status. Low income, poor environmental conditions, inadequate nutrition, and limited access to health, family planning, and medical and social services all combine to make the health of the urban poor very precarious.

Despite the growing problems of the cities, migration from the countryside continues at a rapid pace because of economic and environmental problems in the rural areas and the lure of the real or imagined opportunities in the towns. The average annual growth rate of the urban population in South Asia was 4.0% in 1980–88; in sub-Saharan Africa it was 6.2%. With very few exceptions efforts to curb the movement to the cities in developing countries have failed, and attempts have been made instead to promote planned parenthood and smaller family size.

Fertility

For effective regulation of fertility there needs to be an explicit policy promoting family planning, and this policy needs to be widely known. A further prerequisite is the development of acceptable, accessible, high-quality, family planning services with the public, private, and voluntary sectors working together in partnership. Finally, it is necessary to be able to plan, manage, and monitor these services effectively so as to ensure the appropriate and efficient deployment of scarce resources.

Most developing countries do not have separate population policies for urban and rural areas. However, most governments now consider that the distribution of their populations is unacceptable, and indicates a need to control rapid urban growth.

Most programmes to encourage fertility control tend to be integrated with health programmes, and family planning services are traditionally combined with maternal and child health services. However, in countries where the need to curb population growth is considered to be the highest priority, a separate vertical organization operating in parallel with the district health services may be established. While vertical services may have achieved success in some countries, in general they have been found to be expensive and difficult to manage because they tend to duplicate primary health care services and compete with them for staff and resources.

In a number of countries, duplication and waste have been avoided by having coordinating mechanisms at the highest level of government decision-making—for example, national population commissions at the cabinet or presidential level. At the city level similar coordinating structures may be established.

The promotion of planned parenthood and fertility regulation is greatly helped if it has the support of community leaders and influential people. In many developing countries city-dwellers have set up community and neighbourhood associations for mutual aid and common action. These are found even in slum communities. Where such organizations are directly involved in promoting population control, they usually contribute to the success of the relevant programmes.

The organization of family planning services

Integrated district health systems are particularly effective in promoting fertility regulation. They may be composed of: hospitals, clinics, dispensaries, and mobile units run by a city government; a network of private hospitals, clinics, and industrial medical practitioners; nongovernmental clinics and health facilities run by charitable, religious, and other organizations; and organizations providing health and family planning services for special groups such as trade unions, company workers, civil servants, etc. Because of the great variety of such services in urban areas, collaboration and coordination are particularly important. The concentration in cities of a variety of services concerned with family planning is an advantage in meeting the challenge to improve urban health. So too are some of the other factors that tend to favour lower fertility in cities: higher literacy levels, higher income, better access to the mass media, and higher expectations among women. In general, urban women do have lower fertility rates than their rural sisters, but there is still a long way to go before they reach acceptable levels.

Migrants

In most developing countries internal migration typically accounts for one-third to a half of annual population growth in the cities. Rural–urban migrants have relatively high fertility rates and often retain many of the rural values that place a premium on high fertility. Temporary migrants, or those who live for a time in the towns before returning to the villages, tend to use the services in the towns because of the lack of services in the places they have come from. This can overburden urban facilities, while weakening the government's incentive to improve rural facilities.

Young people

Young people in urban areas tend to be at a disadvantage when it comes to using health and family planning services. One of the main effects of rapid urbanization is the breakdown of the family

24

networks that used to support and protect the young. By the year 2000, half of the world's population will be under 25 years of age and there will be over 500 million young people aged 15–19 needing sex education and family planning services. A substantial proportion of them will be living in the cities of developing countries.

A particularly difficult problem in the cities of developing countries, as in cities everywhere, is the high rate of pregnancy and sexually transmitted disease in teenagers, together with the new threat of HIV infection and AIDS. There is often a lack of services to respond to these problems. In some urban societies, sex education for adolescents remains unknown because of social taboos and religious beliefs. In many developing countries young unmarried adults are generally denied access to contraceptives. The usual reaction when teenage girls become pregnant is to expel them from school, condemning them to a future in which the best they can hope for is an early marriage. Often the unwanted pregnancy is terminated illegally by a backstreet abortionist with the attendant risks to life and health. Three-quarters of maternal deaths in developing countries are due to five main causes, of which illegal abortion is one (the others are haemorrhage, infection, toxaemia, and obstructed labour). The rate of maternal death is twice as high in women aged 15-19 as it is in those aged 20–24, and the first child of a teenage mother is 80% more likely to die than the second or third child of a woman aged 20–24.

Women

The social and economic situation of women in developing areas puts them in a disadvantaged position from the start; in urban areas it may be even worse. Studies of rural–urban migration show that women do not have much say in the decision to move to the town. This is especially the case when migration is related to marriage or the desire to keep the family together, or where the woman is regarded as a dependant.

A particularly alarming trend in many large cities is the rapid growth of households headed by women as a consequence of teenage pregnancy, abandonment by the husband or partner, separation, or divorce. These households are often poor because women find it difficult to combine full-time employment with looking after their children and the home. In many urban areas, the safety net of kinship or the extended family has gone and, even in Bangladesh and India, where the care of widows is one of the main duties of children, the rapid increase in the number of elderly women who have been abandoned is a critical problem.

Although the education of girls has been shown to be one of the most important factors in controlling fertility, their educational level still lags seriously behind that of boys, even in urban areas. This is particularly serious because it has been shown that educational level is directly related to health and well-being.

Chapter 3

Development of urban environmental health services

Urban environmental health is not a new problem. Modern public health was born in the cities of nineteenth-century Europe, when environmental sanitation was used as the major means of controlling infectious diseases, with remarkable effect. For a time, in the aftermath of the Second World War, it was generally believed that therapeutics held the key to future health improvements. As a result, many countries neglected the traditional environmental tasks of public health and, in many of the cities of the developing world which had still to develop a sanitary infrastructure, environmental health was given low priority. However, in recent years public health has once again been on the move. The reasons for this are complex and include the currently dominant political philosophies which oppose increases in publicly funded health and social services and emphasize individual responsibility.

Throughout the 1970s most countries experienced crises in funding public health care systems. The escalating costs were, in part, a consequence of technological innovations in treatment methods, together with an apparently limitless demand for medical care and the rapidly aging populations to be found in many parts of the world. The analysis by the academic Thomas McKeown (2), which seemed to demonstrate that improvements in health in the past had largely been determined by changes in the environment and in lifestyle, and that by Ivan Illich (3), which showed the burden of illness that actually resulted from medical intervention, were two particularly important contributions to the debate. In 1974, the Canadian Government published a report by the then Minister of Health, Marc Lalonde, entitled *A new perspective on the health of Canadians* (4), which focused attention on the fact that a great deal of early death and disability in Canada was avoidable. This report stimulated a multitude of similar reports around the world and was arguably the starting-point for the so-called "new public health".

What has emerged is an approach that combines environmental change and personal preventive measures with appropriate therapeutic interventions, and seeks to get the balance between them right. In the new public health the environment is seen as being social and psychological as well as physical. The Victorian public health movement was constructed round the powerful motivating concept that came to be known as "the sanitary idea"—the idea that overcrowding in insanitary conditions was at the root of the epidemics afflicting the great towns and cities. The application of this idea led to the appointment of City Medical Officers of Health and sanitary inspectors, to departments of public health in local government, and to laws, regulations, and standards for housing, sanitation, water, and food among other things.

Today people are increasingly making the connection between the urban condition and the ecological crisis confronting the planet. The focus on changing lifestyles, which was a preoccupation of industrialized countries in the 1980s, has paved the way for a new concentration on the environment and an understanding of public health based on ecology rather than the more limited and mechanical concept of sanitation. According to the report of the World Commission on Environment and Development (5):

> There are also environmental trends that threaten to radically alter the planet, that threaten the lives of many species upon it, including the human species. Each year another 6 million hectares of productive dryland turns into worthless desert. Over three decades, this would amount to an area roughly as large as Saudi Arabia. More than 11 million hectares of forests are destroyed yearly, and this, over three decades, would equal an area about the size of India. Much of this forest is converted to low-grade farmland unable to support the farmers who settle it. In Europe, acid precipitation kills forests and lakes and damages the artistic and architectural heritage of nations; it may have acidified vast tracts of soil beyond reasonable hope of repair. The burning of fossil fuels puts into the atmosphere carbon dioxide, which is causing gradual global warming. This "greenhouse effect" may by early next century have increased average global temperatures enough to shift agricultural production areas, raise sea levels to flood coastal cities, and disrupt national economies. Other industrial gases threaten to deplete the planet's protective ozone shield to such an extent that the number of human and animal cancers would rise sharply and the oceans' food chain would be disrupted. Industry and agriculture put toxic substances into the human food chain and into underground water tables beyond reach of cleansing.

There is a growing recognition around the world of the need to grapple with the man-made crises that threaten global ecosystems. These crises are, in large part, the result of the lifestyles and expectations of city-dwellers in the way they affect patterns of agriculture and world development, and of our failure to come up with ecologically sound forms of town planning. It is becoming increasingly clear that some of the engineering solutions to the environmental problems of the cities cannot be adequately dealt with using outdated approaches. The ecological idea of understanding how complex natural systems interact and of working with, rather than on, them carries with it at least as great a potential for contributing to human well-being as the sanitary idea did 150 years ago.

A recent workshop of environmental health and public health professionals (6) concluded that four principles should be applied in making an economic appraisal of any city. The first is that town planning, agriculture, and other human interventions should aim as far as possible at working with the natural geographical and biological systems rather than imposing themselves on them. Working with the natural characteristics of an environment has advantages as regards drainage and water supply, ventilation, insulation, indoor climates, and microclimates. It is also desirable from the aesthetic standpoint.

Secondly, diversity and variety should be aimed at in the physical, social, and economic structuring of communities. Land use should be mixed where this does not create hazards. Monolithic housing estates should be a thing of the past, and increasing integration of work, residence, and leisure facilities should reduce the volume of traffic and the danger and pollution associated with it. Thirdly, artificially created systems should be as closed as possible. The application of this principle in environmental management would mean recycling human and solid wastes locally wherever possible and making increased use of renewable sources of water, energy, and raw materials. Lastly, there should be an optimal balance between population and resources. Urban and population change needs to be related to the fragile state of natural systems and the environments that support them.

Effectively there are now two agendas for environmental health in urban areas: the "old" agenda of tackling the basic sanitary problems of large numbers of people who are inadequately housed and often lack a proper water supply and basic sanitation; and the new agenda of dealing with the ecological problems that are rapidly storing up threats to human habitats around the world. These agendas are in effect linked by the lifestyles of urban dwellers. If they are to implement them, the public health departments in most of the world's cities require strengthening.

The task

Urban settlements, from megacities to small towns, are frequently characterized by:

— high population density, overcrowding, congestion, traffic problems, and unsuitable housing;

— large populations living in slums without adequate sanitary provision on sites vulnerable to landslides, floods, and other hazards;

— high levels of environment-related diseases and injuries among increasing numbers of poor people, especially women and children who are particularly exposed to hazards at work and in the home;

— increasing biological, chemical, and physical pollution from industrialization, vehicles, energy production, and the unsatisfactory management of human and solid wastes;

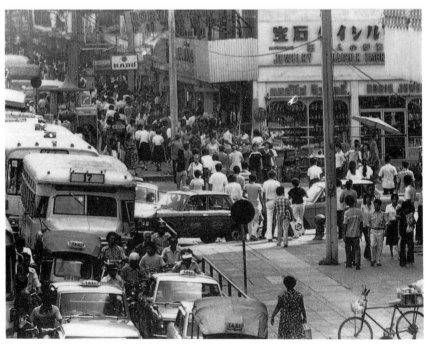

WHO/Zafar (20925)

Rapid urban growth and excessive reliance on the motor car for transport create traffic chaos in cities around the world.

— financial and administrative inability to provide a sanitary infrastructure, coordinate and improve the efficiency of public services, promote employment and housing opportunities, manage wastes, and ensure environmental security.

The environment affects health through such factors as: water supply, domestic and community sanitation, standing surface-water, insect and other vector populations, industrial and residential pollution, working conditions, transport conditions, the quality of housing, the use of chemicals, food supply and food safety, radiation, noise, and the availability of green and open space.

Urbanization is a key factor in sustainable health development

- Urbanization magnifies the effects of mishaps and mismanagement, e.g., breakdowns in water supply and sanitation affect large numbers of people; poor vector control and endemic infectious diseases among the poor threaten the middle classes as well.

- City-dwellers generate large volumes of wastes which can be both directly and indirectly hazardous.

- Urban living is highly interdependent, e.g., much of the food consumed by urban populations is processed and prepared by others, so that effective control of food production, transport, marketing, and handling is needed.

- The effects of natural and man-made disasters are greater in concentrations of population.

- Much urban housing is rented, multiplex, and crowded; the hazards include fire, infectious disease, stress, and domestic pollution.

- Concentrations of buildings and emissions from industrial plants and traffic increase the effects of heat, stress, and air pollution during temperature inversions, while decreasing natural ventilation.

- Cities affect rural areas by increasing the demand for consumer goods, stimulating greater use of agricultural chemicals to meet food needs, increasing pollution, and depleting biomass fuel reserves.

The magnitude of these problems and of their impact on urban health demands a re-examination of environmental health services and a revitalized role for public health services in resolving them.

Environmental health is a social matter

Too often environmental health is seen as a set of compartmentalized activities relating to the physical environment: traditionally, environmental sanitation; more recently, the control of environmental pollutants. The danger of this view is that it fails to see environmental health as an integral part of urban development, with the result that opportunities are missed for promoting behavioural changes that will minimize environmental hazards, bring about sustainable development, and improve the quality of urban life.

When the environment is considered from the point of view of physical and social ecology, effective environmental health action involves much more than the usual legal responsibility for policing the physical infrastructure. Since the protection and promotion of human health are a major goal of the whole of society, environmental health must be concerned with all the individual or organized activities that contribute to the state of the environment and can affect people's health. With this in mind, health authorities can play a more effective role in environmental health. The promotion and protection of public health depends on optimizing the environmental factors that affect it. These include the state of the sanitary infrastructure, the availability of safe food, air pollution levels, and the management of hazardous wastes. Social policy choices can appear to involve trade-offs between competing goals:

- food supply versus the costs of pesticide pollution,

- rising industrial employment versus potential disruption of the ecosystem,

- resource conservation versus current consumption.

The quality of the decisions on such trade-offs and the exploration of ecologically sound alternative options and visions depend on the quality of the information available to the decision-makers and, increasingly, on an informed public debate.

The results of environmental health policies thus depend on measures of various kinds within national and local communities. The role of the health authorities is a crucial one, and ensuring their own active involvement may be the most valuable contribution they can make to the health-for-all strategy. This means not only taking direct action through programmes managed by themselves, but more importantly influencing action by other organizations—the "foreign ministry" role.

It is essential to increase the awareness of politicians, managers, and the public concerning environmental health hazards. Public health leadership can help to optimize the efforts of other agencies in this area by providing technical support and advocating health-promoting choices. For this to be possible, sound "health intelligence" must be available. The role of the health authorities includes defining and assessing health needs and determinants of environmental health; identifying policies that can reduce health problems by countering adverse environmental effects; communicating "health intelligence" to decision-makers in the relevant sectors; and providing technical support for the implementation of policies.

In the public sector, health is affected by activities in the following areas: agriculture (food production, agrochemical use, land-use practices), industry and labour (protection of workers, disposal of wastes, control of emissions), housing and public works, sanitation, transport, education and communications, crime control, social welfare, energy generation, forests and fisheries, and environmental management. Activities in the relevant areas of the private sector also need to be addressed; this may be particularly important when they fall outside the scope of government regulations. Environmental effects on health are often determined by individuals and small groups—for instance, throughout the world mud-house construction is carried out by small-scale enterprises. Local practices in construction, water use, sanitation, waste disposal, and housekeeping can have enormous environmental health consequences. To tackle these issues effectively an intersectoral approach is needed.

How actively and how well national and local health authorities carry out environmental health work depends on their legal obligations, their degree of interest, and their capability. Overall—at the moment universally—the situation is ominous; it is particularly bad in some of the cities with the worst problems.

In many industrialized countries the health authorities have handed environmental health responsibilities over to the ministry of the environment. In developing countries such responsibilities usually remain within the ministry of health, which is generally not equipped to deal with the problems confronting it. Cities in these countries are faced with a massive shortage of technical and monetary resources, insufficient trained manpower, and a lack of environmental health information and intelligence.

33

Health authority functions

Leadership functions

- Advocacy of measures to protect the health of the public
- Fostering the community's capacity for action by encouraging and supporting community self-help programmes
- Carrying out health-impact and risk assessments
- Conducting epidemiological surveillance of environment-related disease

Advisory and participatory functions

- Training personnel to identify, prevent, and control environmental health hazards
- Establishing and operating environmental control programmes and services
- Ensuring preparedness for interagency action in the event of emergency
- Collaborating to develop norms, standards, and legislation
- Carrying out evaluations of the health implications of socio-economic development and planning (environmental health-impact assessments)
- Carrying out research into health-related environmental problems

Targets for environmental health services

Adequate and safe water supply

Safe water is essential to life, hygiene, and the prevention of diarrhoeal and other infectious diseases; water is also needed for industrial and commercial activities that help to improve living standards. The main emphasis in urban water supply programmes in recent decades has been on increasing the provision of piped drinking-water; this emphasis has often overshadowed concern for water quality and safety, water resources, and wastewater management. While the need for adequate water supplies for urban populations cannot be overstated, urban population pressures, industrialization, and increasing environmental constraints mean that water policy needs to be considered from the point of view of sustainable

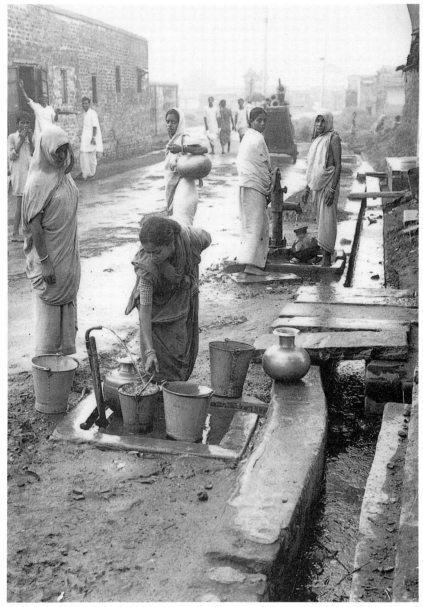

WHO/P. Almasy (7824)

Getting water into households is essential to better health for urban dwellers.

development. The need for water in the cities cannot be met if regional watersheds are depleted and ecosystems disrupted; safeguards against pollution must be maintained if water supplies are not to become agents for the spread of infection and for chronic exposure to harmful substances; the public needs to be considered as a partner in protecting and conserving water supplies and in ensuring their proper use.

Basic sanitation

In most cities in developing countries, the facilities for sewage and wastewater disposal are not as well developed as the water supply facilities; as a result people living in slums and shanty towns face a serious risk of communicable disease. In tropical climates in particular, poor drainage of standing surface-water is an important factor in transmission of infection, both through direct contact and by providing breeding-places for insects that spread particular diseases.

Soil pollution by excreta and biological wastes is also a health hazard, particularly in urban areas where small-scale agriculture is practised.

The disposal of excreta so as not to contaminate surface waters becomes a particular problem as populations grow. Economic factors often limit the extent to which a publicly funded infrastructure can be developed in response to public health needs; however urban communities can help through cooperative and neighbourhood schemes. In recent years, the development of low-cost techniques for basic sanitation has added to the range of practical solutions to such problems. Health education and community organizations are equally important in enabling people to improve sanitary conditions in households and neighbourhoods.

Disposal of solid and hazardous wastes

The management of solid wastes in urban areas becomes more difficult as populations increase and living standards rise; in the latter instance, the increased amounts of domestic and commercial waste that are generated tend to include more non-biodegradable or toxic components. Certain industrial processes also generate toxic residues; the disposal of medical wastes is a particular problem.

Cities in developing countries often lack technical and financial means for the adequate collection, handling, and disposal of solid wastes, and the management of hazardous wastes is a problem in almost every country. Most growing cities have increasing difficulty

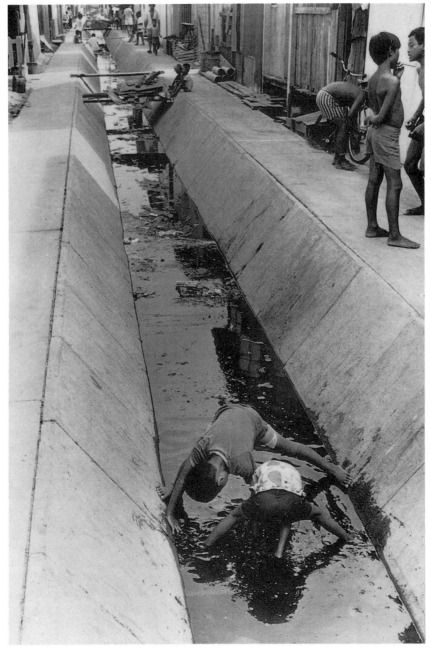

WHO/UNICEF/M. Halevi (20953)

Open drains, a regular feature in low-income urban settlements, represent a major hazard to health.

in finding disposal sites within reasonable distances, while decaying organic matter supports rodent and insect vectors of infectious diseases and water-holding containers encourage insect-breeding. Refuse dumps present the risk of toxic exposure and may leak into ground and surface waters; incineration can pollute the air with particulates and organically active chemicals.

In addition to systematic waste collection, a many-sided approach to the problem is needed; we are a long way from the ecological production and management of wastes in most urban areas of the world. There is a need to reduce the amount of waste generated by shifting to reusable materials, using biodegradable packaging, and planning for much more recovery and recycling, composting, and compacting. Public education on waste reduction and on proper handling and storage is also needed to minimize the risks of disease and injury. The management of hazardous wastes requires proficiency in the identification, assessment, and monitoring of hazards; the setting and enforcement of standards; modification of the processes employed and safe disposal methods; the cleaning-up of abandoned waste sites; and public education and information.

Control of air and water pollution

Industrial processes, power production, and personal transport in urban areas are the main causes of air pollution. The resulting environmental and health effects differ: for example, tropical cities are more likely to suffer from photochemical smog, while children are more susceptible to lead pollution than adults.

Problems of indoor air pollution vary, depending on climate. In tropical countries, health problems can arise from the burning of biomass fuels in poorly ventilated houses. In colder climates, where people spend more time indoors and buildings are designed to minimize the exchange of indoor and outdoor air, pollutants may be trapped inside homes and workplaces and reach dangerous levels. Major sources of water pollution include the insanitary disposal of excreta and collected sewage, leaking waste dumps, and discharges of industrial effluent and mining waste. Other sources of chemical pollution are improperly managed agrochemicals, airborne particles and fumes, biotic changes resulting from large-scale water resource developments, and spillage of chemicals in fresh water and sea water during transport. Preventing and dealing with environmental pollution needs skills in identifying and assessing hazards, establishing standards and regulations, designing and implementing controls, monitoring problem situations, and enforcing norms. Public educa-

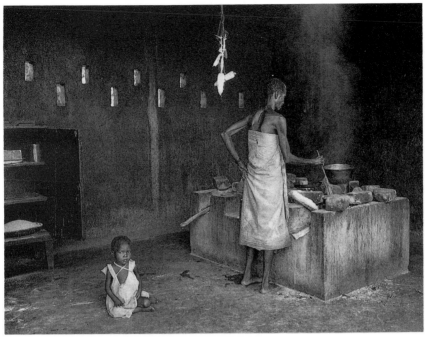

WHO/C. Stauffer (20648)

Chimney-less fireplaces are a source of indoor air pollution and a permanent health hazard for many families in developing countries.

tion and the promotion of "primary environmental care" are necessary. Pollution control must involve the collaboration of many agencies and organizations, and there is a particular need for intergovernmental collaboration to deal with pollution in cities that are downstream to numerous contributory sources.

Chemical safety

The increased use of chemicals in industry, agriculture, and food processing, and in the home, means that controls are now needed to reduce acute and long-term exposure to health-damaging substances, and to prevent and deal with chemical accidents that may have widespread effects. The risks are extensive, affecting people involved in chemical production and distribution, users of chemical products in industry, commerce, agriculture, and the home, and populations exposed to accidental spillages. Control programmes tend to be particularly weak in developing countries,

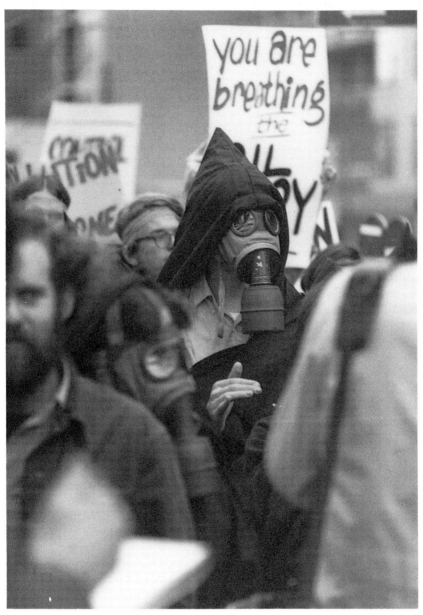

WHO/J. Mohr (15406)

Public opinion—epitomized by these young demonstrators in New York—is increasingly aware of the potential dangers of chemical pollution.

and the importation of certain chemicals that are banned in industrialized countries makes the situation worse. Although the increasing use of agrochemicals creates real hazards in rural areas, the concentration of populations in towns and cities makes chemical safety a significant environmental health problem in urban areas too.

Food safety

Traditional efforts to protect consumers against the microbial contamination of food now need to be extended to deal with the problems created by pesticide residues and the substances used in food preservation, as well as the risk of animal foodstuffs suffering environmental contamination. Further potential problems are posed by the extensive consumption of "fast food" and convenience foods, which is largely an urban phenomenon. People on low incomes in urban areas are at particular risk of eating spoiled and improperly prepared food. Throughout the world there is a need for better integration of programmes for food and chemical safety and the control of environmental pollution. There is a particular need in many cities to strengthen services for the marketing, handling, and preparation of food, notably by improving the training of food-handlers.

Occupational safety

Industries in urban areas tend to make use of relatively advanced technologies and untried processes. These carry with them increased risks both for workers and for the surrounding populations.

In developing countries, legislation to protect workers may be weak or non-existent; so too may standards or enforcement. Protection is even weaker for the increasing number of workers in the informal economy, who are seldom represented by labour organizations or recognized by official regulators. New migrants to cities may be at a particular disadvantage in being unaware of their rights or unacquainted with safe working practices. Where city health authorities do not have direct responsibility for occupational health and safety, they can play an active role in this area through advocacy and monitoring and by acting as convenors of the various groups with an interest in protecting public health.

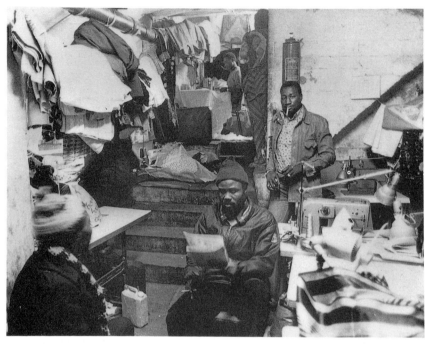

WHO/J. Mohr (20960)

Cottage industry is a major employer in many cities, especially for newcomers or people without access to the formal employment sector, but is often associated with long hours, poor pay, and inadequate or non-existent provisions for occupational safety.

Accident and disaster prevention and control

The concentration of people, industry, and traffic in urban areas creates conditions in which disasters are not only more likely, but apt to be more serious than in rural areas. Residents of squatter settlements in flood-prone areas and on unsuitable hillside sites are highly vulnerable; accidents contribute substantially to mortality and morbidity in children, while traffic accidents in particular are a leading cause of death and disability among adolescents and young adults. Health authorities can be actively involved in environmental and behaviour-modifying measures to prevent accidents and disasters due to human negligence, and in ensuring that the emergency services to deal with them are adequate. Close interorganizational collaboration is required to ensure effective action in the event of a disaster.

42

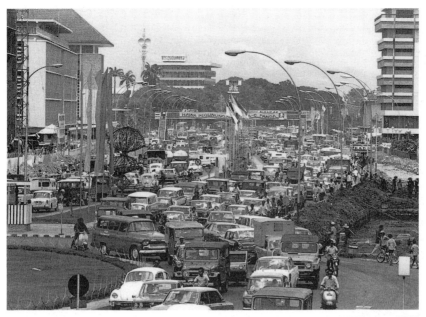

WHO/J. Mohr (16533)

Reaching the limits? Heavy traffic clogs a street in Jakarta, Indonesia.

Taking an integrated approach

Although it is conventional to describe environmental health in terms of different categories and tasks, the environmental components of public health can be most effectively dealt with by approaching them in a systematic and integrated way. The desired integration can best be achieved by:

— reorienting environmental health services to deal with different hazards as part of an overall health development strategy;

— establishing environmental health priorities based on cost-effectiveness and on the potential health gains for the population;

— formulating short- and long-term plans that include specific targets to be achieved within defined time periods and involve collaboration between different agencies and organizations;

— organizing coordinated monitoring and evaluation with appropriate criteria and indicators to assess progress towards health targets.

Strengthening environmental health services in cities

Public health departments in most of the world's cities need strengthening if the urban environment is to support rather than undermine the health of its inhabitants. Their traditional environmental health functions in developing (and some developed) countries are centred on the control of infectious and communicable diseases. Typically they are concerned with the inspection of public eating-places, the examination and licensing of food handlers, and advisory and enforcement work in some aspects of housing hygiene—functions that are often perceived by the public, especially in developing countries, as indicating a "police" role fraught with the danger of possible penalties. If involved at all in pollution control, their main function is limited to providing information on criteria and standards.

Public health departments may suffer from a low status compared with other city departments, and environmental health units within a public health department may be accorded a low status. These units are frequently understaffed, consisting mainly of sanitary inspectors.

A more effective public health presence is needed. The health aspects of shelter, transport, employment, food and water supply, and toxic waste are key issues in the cities, and environmental health services that address these areas are becoming even more necessary as city populations expand. It is particularly important for city health departments to become actively involved in health promotion and in the monitoring and control of the whole range of environmental hazards. The challenge is to meet both the old sanitary agenda and the new ecological one and to see that activities are fully integrated with primary health care at the neighbourhood level. The leadership role of the public health authority is crucial; first of all, because this authority is usually responsible for taking an overview of the health of the whole population. Secondly, it is commonly seen as having no vested interest other than a legitimate concern for human health whenever there is any question of setting economic and environmental development against possible adverse effects on health.

Strengthening environmental health can be a powerful strategy for protecting health in the context of sustainable development. Taking the health consequences of development into account and making sure that prevention has a seat at the table are priority issues. To realize the potential for health gains in this way, a deliberate strategy for environmental health must be formulated within the framework of economic and health development.

> Ministries of health can support local environmental health services in urban areas by:
>
> — providing health information to those concerned with the management of environmental health activities;
>
> — linking environmental data with health status in order to assist various agencies, such as those dealing with housing, water, and sanitation, to support and promote health;
>
> — focusing on occupational health as a specific, often neglected, aspect of environmental health;
>
> — carrying out population surveys to find out the degree of public satisfaction with the environmental health services.

The need for political support

Overall there is a need for politicians to be more aware of environmental issues and of the interrelationships between development, health, and the environment. There is a need for political commitment to the development of environmental health services and to ensuring that health and environmental health are incorporated in urban development plans. The need for ministries of health to support local environmental action has implications for the training of health personnel and for their endowment with the relevant concepts, attitudes, and skills.

Although urban environmental health departments need to change the way they work, they still have to focus clearly on some ever-present public health threats, including vector-borne diseases such as malaria, filariasis, and others that thrive in urban areas. In all environmental health matters, leadership is of the greatest importance, and health workers need to accept the new styles of working needed, for example, in facilitating community initiatives. Physicians, engineers, nurses, managers, and other health workers need to develop partnerships at the neighbourhood level to work for improved environmental conditions. This process can be assisted by the decentralization of responsibilities.

A number of studies have shown women's central role in community initiatives. Unfortunately, there is usually an imbalance between what they put in and how they benefit personally, as well as a large gap between the training and resources available to men and those available to women.

45

Chapter 4

Reorienting the urban health system

The increasing drive for a new public health movement to tackle the problems of the twenty-first century has been reflected in numerous WHO meetings and in such texts as the Declaration of Alma-Ata (7) and the Global Strategy for Health for All by the Year 2000 (8). WHO has incorporated their main principles in its Healthy Cities Project.

The focus is on the situation of the poor and disadvantaged, the need to reorient medical services and health systems away from hospital care and towards primary health care, the importance of public involvement and of an effective partnership between the public, private, and voluntary sectors. The concept of health promotion, which restates the importance of public policy and environmental action as well as individual behavioural changes, has been influential in the move from an individualistic, victim-blaming approach to one that identifies the environmental and organizational measures needed to support public health. It is unlikely that there can be standard packaged solutions to the problems of city life and health, except possibly with regard to their more technical aspects. It therefore seems appropriate to consider the urban health system as including all the social and economic factors affecting health status, whether in the public, private, or voluntary sector.

The urban district health system

The health district is the most peripheral fully organized unit of local government and administration. It differs greatly from country to country, both in size and in the degree of autonomy it enjoys. As a unit it is small enough for the staff to understand the major problems and constraints of socioeconomic and health development, but large enough for the development of the technical and managerial skills essential for the effective running of an integrated system. The district is the natural meeting-point for "bottom–up" planning and organization and "top–down" planning and support, and is therefore a place where community needs and national priorities are most appropriately reconciled. The urban district, often with its own political mandate and highly developed sense of local identity and pride, is in a unique position to tackle major public health problems and to enlist the involvement of various sectors, driven by a combination of enlightened self-interest and a sense of belonging and commitment to the city.

In WHO's strategy for health for all by the year 2000 (8), primary health care is put forward as the method whereby this goal may be achieved. There are, in fact, four ways in which primary health care can be interpreted:

- as a set of activities
- as a level of care
- as a strategy for organizing health care
- as a philosophy.

The eight activities identified as the basic elements of primary health care in the Declaration of Alma-Ata can be taken as the most down-to-earth starting-point:

— health education

— food supply and proper nutrition

— safe water and basic sanitation

— maternal and child health care

— immunization

— prevention and control of endemic disease

— basic treatment of health problems

— provision of essential drugs.

These activities need to be seen in the light of two imperatives: concern for social justice, and understanding of their ecological impact. The health of the most disadvantaged and poorest groups in big cities is deteriorating relative to that of the better-off, and this will continue to be a growing cause of concern with accelerating urbanization. The urban rich have a major responsibility for meeting the needs of the urban poor. There are both moral and pragmatic reasons for this. The moral reason ought to be self-evident and should be considered in the light of the major philosophical and

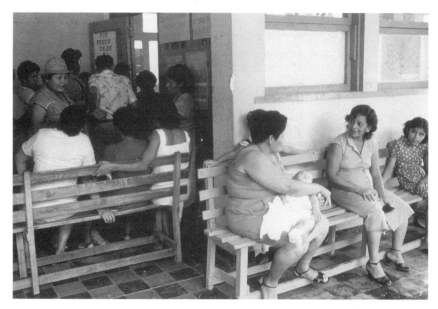

Urban health centres, offering a range of health promotion, preventive medicine and treatment services, are the basis of an effective urban district health system.

religious movements of the world that provide social cohesion and stability. At a pragmatic level and from the perspective of enlightened self-interest, the consequences of not addressing these issues will affect all city-dwellers in that there is little respect for wealth or status in the spread of disease and violence and the reduction in the quality of city life.

The district health system based on primary health care is seen by many people as the key to tackling these issues. This system is a more or less self-contained segment of the national health system. It comprises a well-defined population living within a clearly delineated administrative and geographical area. It includes all the relevant health care personnel and facilities in the area, such as health posts, dispensaries, health centres, and hospitals, governmental or otherwise, together with laboratory, diagnostic, and other supporting services. It therefore consists of a great variety of interrelated elements that contribute to health in homes, schools, workplaces, communities, and the health sector and related social and economic sectors. The district health system will be most effective if coordinated by an appropriately trained director of public health, working to ensure as comprehensive a range as possible of promotive, preventive, curative, and rehabilitative activities. Although it is necessary for somebody to have an overview of the health of the population of the city, there is no need for the city itself to attempt to provide all the services that might be desired in response to the health problems identified. It is necessary to distinguish between means and ends, and public health leadership may be made most effective through the provision of information, norm-setting, monitoring, and enforcement, in addition to those direct services whose provision is regarded as a core public health function.

There are four main factors to be considered in ensuring that a district health system adequately addresses the population's health needs:

— access

— quality and information

— financing

— accountability.

Access

A public health imperative is that of population coverage irrespective of social position. The main problem with urban health care is not simply that it lacks quality and comprehensiveness but that, because of maldistribution of facilities, it is often not easily accessible to those in need.

A comprehensive programme of primary health care for poor urban areas would include: generating employment through collaboration with other sectors; improving the efficiency of food distribution through support for food shops and community gardens; and providing support for owner-built housing and sanitation. The health sector would participate in the development of policies for systems of education, and initiatives in other areas of everyday life, including the provision of energy and public transport. For a city to begin to tackle its problems, a social contract is needed in which the better-off accept responsibility for enabling the poor to have access to essential services. However, this does not mean that everything needs to be done for, and to, poor communities, and the importance of community involvement in the determination of local priorities and concerted action cannot be overstated. Many of the resources for improving sanitation, nutrition, or antenatal care can be found within the community itself, and harnessing them will result in better health for the community as a whole. Moreover, communities are more likely to value and look after services to which they have contributed.

One problem is that community participation and community organization in any form are still not politically acceptable in some countries. There is a need for politicians, local government officers, and professionals to accept and support the part to be played by the voluntary sector.

Members of the community can be trained to become community health workers and volunteers, and the community can contribute labour for the construction of health facilities, building materials being provided free or on credit by the government or nongovernmental organizations. Poor communities in both developing and industrialized cities will work to build roads, schools, and clinics, and to organize rubbish and sewage disposal, if they are supported by appropriate policies. Women frequently play a central part in community development initiatives, and they should be encouraged and supported in this. However, community participation implies more than contributing labour—it also requires active involvement and substantial control over planning and implementation.

One essential approach to the improvement of urban services is to develop a wholehearted commitment to decentralization and local integration. To develop and sustain a truly decentralized system, while at the same time insisting on strategic action, requires political determination and vision. Political will is often the major factor in determining whether issues relating to the urban poor are tackled effectively.

Quality and information

Quality standards must be met from the point of view of all three partners in the urban public health task—the public, the professionals, and the paymasters. The shortage of data relevant to health policy is a major weakness in many cities. Even quite basic environmental and personal health data can be of considerable help in targeting resources and monitoring the impact of policies and interventions.

There has so far been only limited progress in developing operationally useful measurements of the outcome of health action, even in the most generously funded systems, and techniques for monitoring the quality of services, such as peer audit, still lack widespread acceptance. There is an urgent need for political commitment to ensuring that the monitoring and evaluation of urban health systems are combined with an understanding of what is good practice. This has significant implications for the training of all professional health care and social workers. Making such data as exist available in an accessible form is a powerful and effective way of mobilizing community leaders and securing their involvement in community organizations to solve health problems. At the more sophisticated level of data collection and analysis, there are weaknesses in the scientific basis of health risk assessment—for example, with regard to the effect of chronic low-level exposures to pollution and the combined and synergistic effects of toxic substances. There is a need to support the development of environmental and ecological epidemiology to clarify the adverse and beneficial impacts of urban conditions on mental and physical health. It is important for research on health status to include surveys of health and environmental conditions in poor communities and for differences in health status to be measured in different parts of a city. The use of citywide averages often hides enormous variations between neighbourhoods. Such data can enable planners to put forward policies for more equitable distribution of resources.

A particular problem is that it can be difficult even to determine who lives in the poorest neighbourhoods of the city, because of homelessness, lack of secure legal status, and the unstructured nature of many settlements. When areas are not legally recognized and when people are suspicious of authority, official information will be very hard to obtain. Information about health needs and the results of health action should be both objective, using quantified indicators such as literacy levels, mortality and morbidity rates, and sanitation provision, and subjective, taking account of people's opinions about their difficulties and their needs. Information about disease, health, and the quality of life can be a major driving-force for change. The little information that is currently available is often not used effectively to fuel the dialogue that should take place between politicians, managers, health care professionals, and the public about the most appropriate services and their location. There is a need for appropriate local "shoe leather" epidemiology and the aggregation of information to different levels for different purposes. There is a particular need to try to anticipate changing health needs and to predict trends for the future, particularly as regards age and sex balance. Good basic health information should be seen as a resource and not as an unnecessary expense. There is a need to develop a shared agenda, based on real information, between the public and the health workers and to raise public awareness with the help of the media, educational institutions, and cultural and social centres.

Ten questions based on those used in the Pan American Health Organization's Healthy Communities Initiative[a]

1. Is there an analysis of the main health problems and conditions in each part of the main urban areas and at each stage of life?

2. Is this information widely available in cities so that people are able to discuss what needs to be done to improve health?

3. Do people have access to information about what health services are available and how to get access to them as needed?

4. Is action being taken to create safer, healthier, and ecologically sound physical and social environments that will support healthier lifestyles in urban areas?

5. Are all areas of everyday life—public, private, and voluntary—involved in planning and working for better urban health?

6. Is there an effective way of getting everybody to work together at the neighbourhood level?

7. Are there mechanisms for identifying and supporting community leaders who speak out for better health and make sure that the factors that affect health are understood by the public? Do the city hospitals provide public health leadership?

8. Do cities have specific plans to collect and distribute needed information about health, to develop stronger intersectoral cooperation, and to provide adequate resources for health?

9. Is it necessary to establish new organizational infrastructures to facilitate an integrated approach to urban health, or can existing structures be adapted and made to work?

10. Is there a clear understanding and consensus regarding the relative contributions of central and local government to the improvement and protection of urban health?

[a] *Working together towards health for all. Healthy communities for the Americas.* Washington, DC, PAHO, 1988.

Examples of population-based and territorially based data on primary health care are reported from a number of countries. Such data seem to be more easily obtainable where community health workers are well integrated into both the health care and social care systems, and where health posts or clinics maintain comprehensive records on the defined population they serve. Where systematic information-gathering does not exist, novel approaches to the measurement of health status may be possible. These include the use of sentinel families or neighbourhoods, audits of the care of patients brought in dead to hospital, and comparisons of absenteeism due to illness among schoolchildren from different parts of the city.

A major contemporary trend in health care throughout the world is the move away from a monolithic organizational and monodisciplinary approach to one that depends on strategic situation analysis, option appraisal, and multiple varied interventions. With the newer approach, it is essential that responsibility for taking an overview of the quality of health systems should rest with an identified individual such as a director of public health.

Financing

The level of resources available to any urban health system depends on a political decision unique to the place concerned. However, the way in which the available resources are distributed raises fundamental questions about social justice. The concentration of populations in urban areas can bring health benefits in the form of variety of response and economy of scale. On the other hand urban areas that are out of control can experience a vicious cycle of environmental degradation, crime, and physical and social ill-health. This can be difficult to break out of, in the absence of concerted central political action and the injection of resources.

If funding levels cannot be raised, cities need to find the most effective way of re-allocating existing resources to release other human and capital resources available for health within the population. When material resources are available, the emphasis should be on mobilizing them to improve the physical infrastructure for health, through investment in such areas as sanitation and safe water supplies.

Fund-raising by committees and through charity and self-help groups can play an important part in providing additional resources for primary health care, as can the development of health insurance through non-profit-making organizations such as friendly societies or through compulsory insurance schemes. Recent experience with user charges for health services indicates that their introduction discourages the poor from using services.

Accountability

The extent to which urban health systems are accountable to the populations they serve varies enormously, as does the responsibility of cities for the provision of primary health care. A general problem in cities throughout the world is failure to take an overview of all the factors affecting health and to devise mechanisms to ensure that all the relevant agencies and organizations are pulling in the same direction. The need for closer intersectoral collaboration is apparent everywhere, and the establishment of some kind of interagency coordinating committee at the highest level and chaired by the city mayor is now frequently advocated.

The "horizontal" problems of lack of interagency and interorganizational integration are frequently made worse by the "vertical" problems of lack of integration with community initiatives, on the one hand, and government initiatives, on the other. It is now common to find a demand both for the strengthening and reform of local government and for a clarification of the relationships between local and national administrations. Where a city has no overall plan for health development, it is important that it should be encouraged to move towards one. However, the preparation of such a plan is not an end in itself but a means to an end. The process of debate and discussion surrounding the development of a plan can help motivate members of the general public to join community organizations working to improve health. Other approaches that have been found useful in encouraging public involvement include neighbourhood workshops and twinning and exchange schemes permitting citizens with common interests from different cities to exchange experiences and learn from each other.

Changing urban health systems

Although health services and other forms of investment in health care tend to be heavily concentrated in the cities, there is a mismatch between the services available and those that would be most effective with the limits of the resources available. For example:

— Acute hospitals, which are intended for patients referred for sophisticated treatments, tend to be used as a point of first contact; this is an inefficient way of using expensive, specialized facilities and can lead to their becoming over-whelmed.

— Services tend to be poorest in the areas where people need them most.

— The emphasis on treatment over the past 30–40 years has tended to leave preventive, first contact, and chronic care services lagging behind.

Because of the gravity of the urban crisis and because of the shortage of resources, it would be wholly impracticable to develop and build a new system side-by-side with the existing one. Leaving existing services as they are is not an option. The reorientation of urban health systems towards health promotion, primary health care, and community-based care in line with the health-for-all strategy seems to be the best way forward. Demographic pressure, combined with shortages of resources and the overloading of the hospital sector, is increasingly leading to experiments with extended forms of primary health care. One example is the elaborated health centre with an extended range of activities; however, it is considered that, for such centres to be successful, their credibility with local populations must be improved. New low-cost technologies and changing patterns of morbidity, with increasing numbers of patients suffering from chronic conditions, have made this kind of development compatible with high quality care. The involvement of hospital doctors in primary health care centres lends credibility to their activities and further relieves pressure on hospital inpatient and outpatient departments. Not infrequently, such centres have evolved from what were originally maternal and child health or family planning clinics.

The range of services available in these centres, known as reference health centres, is wide and is dependent on local traditions, organizational culture, and levels of funding. Typically, they integrate health promotion, preventive medicine, primary health care, and maternal and child health services with the provision of outpatient and day surgery care, specialized treatments being provided by visiting hospital specialists.

This approach seems capable of significantly changing the style and content of hospital services in urban areas in both developing and developed countries, and of facilitating the reorientation of medical care. In special circumstances a reference health centre may also be suitable for delivering health services in a well populated rural area.

Typically, in addition to health promotion, health education, preventive, and primary health care services, the extended range of services in a reference health centre comprises:

- maternal and child health, including family planning and services related to reproductive health

- environmental health services

- general medical care

- community-based nursing and social care

- outpatient services, including day surgery, urgent care of minor injuries, emergency treatment, diagnostic procedures, and rehabilitation

- short-stay inpatient care

- services for underserved and other special groups, including the elderly.

Leadership, organization, and management

The revolution required in health systems and other urban services will not take place by itself. Leadership, organization, and management are not optional extras. However, the appropriate skills are in short supply in many countries, both developed and developing. Cities are not all the same, and there are no ready-made solutions for all their problems. Yet somebody must be responsible for taking an integrated overview of the health situation and for steering health strategy.

The question arises as to who should provide the leadership and whether the person needs to be a doctor. This may be an artificial question, because the leadership needed in deprived and underserved urban areas is likely to be earned on merit rather than endowed by appointment. It needs to be visionary but hard-headed, and at the same time facilitative, and may come from various quarters. However, the changes needed in urban health systems cannot be realized without the active involvement of at least some city doctors. There is a need to change medical education and training so that doctors will be better equipped to work in partnership with other professions and with community groups, and to ensure that the horizontal integration of medical and social care, together with the vertical integration of primary, secondary, and tertiary care, can become a reality.

Universities, medical schools, and other academic institutions have a particular opportunity to demonstrate their relevance by becoming involved with their local communities in pioneering effective urban health systems. Before any urban health strategy can work, it is necessary to resolve basic questions concerning the role of government, the reorientation of local organizations, and the interface between government services and community action. At the moment many public health departments which should be providing leadership are extremely weak. They need political support to ensure that their leadership role is accepted, understood, and strengthened.

Despite difficulties, some cities have shown that imaginative activities can have a major effect on health, especially in the case of the disadvantaged. Examples include:

— training in basic business methods for people starting small businesses or operating in the informal sector;

— help with food distribution to reduce food prices, which tend to be highest in some of the poorest neighbourhoods;

— provision of low-cost building materials and help with securing sites for those wanting to build their own homes;

— support for the organization of refuse collection and processing in slum areas.

Urban and rural areas are interdependent. An effective urban strategy must seek to maintain the prosperity of the surrounding rural areas and the attractiveness of living in them, and to increase the strength of the rural health care system. The urban district health system has a direct interest in promoting these objectives, if only to take some of the pressure off the urban services.

Strengthening the capacity of the urban health system

The task facing city governments is enormous, and there is no particular relationship between the scale of the situation and the capacity for tackling it. Some of the city administrations where the combination of issues to be tackled is worst are among the most fragile. Real and effective strengthening of the capacity of urban health systems requires an emphasis on community resources as well as on community needs. This presents a challenge to the view held by many health workers that the public are passive consumers of care rather than partners in maintaining and improving health. It is also necessary to find new ways of assessing community capabilities as a first step in mobilizing them for the common good.

An important aspect of the orientation and motivation of health workers is the impact of materialistic as compared with vocational motivation. It seems likely that a rampant free-market philosophy can undermine vocational motivation. On the other hand, in most cities the private and informal sectors are resources that it would be a mistake to ignore. The process of local capacity-building must be carried out at all levels and with all sectors, and must be a continuous one. It needs to involve schools, universities, and other training and research institutions whose work is often not grounded in the social needs of the surrounding populations. With few exceptions efforts to build up the capacity of urban health systems are weak and uncoordinated, and ignore the need for an interdisciplinary and intersectoral approach. The universities and other institutions providing training and research are in a favourable position to support the development of human resources and to enable questions of policy to be addressed in a practical and effective way.

Chapter 5

City networks for health

Many national governments have now committed themselves to working towards health for all as an explicit social goal. In the terms of the Global Strategy for Health for All by the Year 2000 (*8*), this requires a commitment to public participation and to inter-sectoral action aimed at improving health, particularly in the poorest sections of the community. In a rapidly urbanizing world, there also needs to be a clear commitment to this approach on the part of towns and cities and their administrations. The city is often at the lowest level of administration that can marshal the resources and has the political mandate and authority to develop and implement multisec-toral approaches to health; and, because it is a place with which its inhabitants identify, it offers good prospects for obtaining the participation of the public by invoking neighbourhood or civic pride. On this understanding, networks of cities have been de-veloped in all parts of the world in recent years. Such networks may be formed for a variety of purposes—for example, the Metropolis City Network was formed to promote urban development and housing, environmental protection, urban transport, the urban eco-nomy, urban management, and urban health; the United Nations Economic and Social Commission for Asia and the Pacific developed its CITYNET network to promote better urban management; and the European Region of WHO developed its Healthy Cities Project to encourage cities to share experience in health promotion.

City networks can provide the following benefits:

— the sharing of information between members;

— the sharing of resources to solve joint problems, for ex-ample, by developing effective urban management policies;

— the joint development of standards and codes for urban policies and management practices, more or less obliging all members of the network to adopt them, rather than be the odd one out;

— the establishment of a force to influence national and international policies and norms so as to promote healthy urban development. Such a force can, for example, encourage the decentralization of urban management functions and decision-making from national government to municipal government level, this being essential to permit local participation in urban development.

The origins of city-based health initiatives

The idea that the city might be a suitable base on which to build a public health movement is not a new one. In nineteenth-century Europe and North America, the rapid growth of industrial towns and cities created conditions under which epidemic disease was rife, and it was the cities that responded to the challenge.

On 11 December 1844, at a public meeting at Exeter Town Hall in England, the Health of Towns Association was formed at the instigation of the local mayor with the specific purpose of collecting information about health conditions among those living in poor urban areas and of using this information as a basis for change (9). Following that first meeting in Exeter, branches of the Association were formed in twelve of the country's largest towns and cities within a matter of months. Acting in concert, these branches played a significant role in bringing about the sanitary movement of the late 1840s and the 1850s which tackled the public health issues of the day through legislation, environmental improvements, and organizational development.

The Healthy Cities Project developed by the WHO Regional Office for Europe seeks to bring together political and community leaders, local citizens, community organizations, professional associations, and national and international agencies in a collaborative, intersectoral, and community-based effort to achieve health for all at the local level. Networks and coalitions have been established within and between cities, nationally and internationally, and between cities and national and international agencies. The project began with a meeting of representatives of 21 European cities in Lisbon in 1986, who agreed to collaborate in developing sound approaches to the promotion of urban health. It has five major components:

— the formulation of concepts leading to the adoption of action-based city plans for health, using the health-for-all strategy, health promotion principles, and WHO's health targets as a framework (*10*);

— the development of models of good practice representing a variety of different approaches, the choice of which will depend on the perceived priorities and which may range from major environmental action to programmes designed to support changes in individual lifestyles, but should always illustrate the key principles of health promotion;

— monitoring of, and research into, the effects of models of good practice on health in cities.

— the dissemination of ideas and experiences among collaborating cities and other cities that may be interested;

— mutual support, collaboration, and learning and cultural exchanges between European towns and cities.

The participating cities agreed to undertake seven specific tasks:

1. To establish, within each city, a high-level intersectoral group bringing together executive decision-makers from the city's main agencies and organizations. The purpose of the group is to take a strategic overview of health in the city and promote collaboration at every level between the organizations concerned.

2. To establish, as a "shadow" to the executive group, an intersectoral officer or technical group to work on collaborative analysis and planning for health in the city.

3. To carry out a community diagnosis for the city down to the smallest neighbourhood, with an emphasis on inequalities in health and the integration of data from a variety of sources, including an assessment of the public's image of their communities and their personal health.

4. To establish sound working links between the municipality and local educational institutions at both the school and higher education levels. Links at the school level can be explored as partnerships for learning, those at the higher education level as partnerships for research and teaching. The latter links should not be confined to medical training establishments but should extend to any department or institution with an interest in urban health-related phenomena. Part of this work involves the

61

identification of appropriate urban health indicators and targets on the basis of the Barcelona criteria (*11*):

— that they should be sensitive to change in the short term, comparable between cities, and politically visible in order to stimulate change;
— that they should be simple to collect, use, and understand, and should be either directly available now or available in a reasonable time at an acceptable cost;
— that they should be related to health promotion.

5. To ask all sectors to review the health promotion potential of their activities and organizations, and to develop health impact statements as a way of making explicit this potential in different policy areas. This requirement recognizes that within a city there are many untapped health resources, both human and material.

6. To promote a full-scale debate about health within each city, with the free involvement of the public and the active collaboration of the local media. This task might require the encouragement of debate and dialogue using, for example, such points of contact with the public as schools, community centres, museums, libraries, and art galleries. A city's own public health history is in itself a powerful focus for debate and learning. The exploration of ways of developing effective health advocacy at the city level is part of this task.

7. To adopt specific health improvement measures based on the principles of health for all, and to monitor and evaluate these measures. The sharing of experience between cities and the development of cultural links and exchanges is fundamental to this task, which is designed to fulfil one of WHO's basic aims, namely the promotion of world peace and understanding, without which the health of everyone is threatened.

The emphasis in these tasks is on the development of enabling mechanisms for health promotion through sound public policy and increased public accountability; they also aim at breaking down vertical structures and barriers and obtaining much better horizontal integration for joint action. Initiated by WHO's Regional Office for Europe in Copenhagen, the Healthy Cities Project is promoted by the Department of Public Health at the University of Liverpool, England, and the Nordic School of Public Health in Göteborg, Sweden, and is supported by an international newsletter produced in Liverpool. This approach underlines the project's commitment to

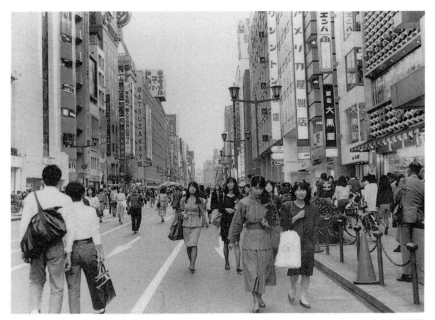

WHO/Zafar (20913)

Shutting out the cars from selected areas is a major innovation for many cities that have developed attractive and popular, pollution-free and safe pedestrian plazas.

reorienting existing institutions and encouraging their involvement at the local level, rather than establishing new organizational forms that duplicate existing arrangements.

By putting health on the social and political agenda of local government, the Healthy Cities Project has (1) made it easier for municipal authorities to develop sound public policies, (2) encouraged urban environmental health services to address not only pollution control but also the wider issues of sustainable development, and (3) promoted the reorientation of urban health services. Because of its commitment to community and local government accountability, the project has also sought to enable people to have increased control over their health and improve it. The apparent success of this approach can be judged by the fact that what was originally intended to be a small-scale project in a few cities has mushroomed to become a project involving 31 cities in Europe; it has been adopted spontaneously on a large scale, and many other national and international networks of cities are now using the same approach. The Healthy Cities Project was at first confined to the developed countries where it originated. More recently, a number of cities in

63

developing countries have become interested in it, and ministers of health of a number of developing countries have recommended "extending the concept of the Healthy Cities Project of Europe to become a worldwide programme" (*11*). It seems likely that the European project will need to be adapted to the particular circumstances of cities in developing countries in various parts of the world, although the underlying philosophy of health for all and its local interpretation have general applicability.

Characteristics of a healthy city

The characteristics of a healthy city are:

- a clean and safe physical environment of high quality (including quality of housing);
- a stable ecosystem that is sustainable in the long term;
- a strong, mutually supportive, and non-exploitative community;
- a high degree of participation and control by the public over the decisions affecting their lives, health, and well-being;
- the meeting of basic needs (for food, water, shelter, income, safety, and work) for all the city's people;
- access to a wide variety of experiences and resources, with extensive opportunity for contact, interaction, and communication;
- a diverse, vital, and innovative urban economy;
- the encouragement of connectedness with the past, with the cultural and biological heritage of the city's inhabitants, and with other groups and individuals;
- an urban layout that is compatible with, and enhances, the preceding characteristics;
- an optimum level of appropriate public health and care services, accessible to all;
- high health status (high levels of positive health and low levels of disease).

Chapter 6

Urban policies for health development

The issues

Relatively few countries have comprehensive national policies on urban development, and most lack the resources and organizational mechanisms needed to produce them. Both the vertical separation between governmental and nongovernmental levels of organization and the horizontal separation between sectors limit the feasibility of introducing coherent policies and programmes.

In general, the more serious constraints arise from poor horizontal or intersectoral linkages. In many countries an urban policy is no more than a patchwork of sectoral policies—for land use, economic development, housing, pollution control, traffic, etc. When major responsibilities are assigned to different levels—for example, when economic development is administered at the national level and land-use planning at local level—difficulties in coordination are increased. It is time-consuming and difficult to integrate intersectoral action, when each sector is organized in the way considered most suitable for its own particular mission. Countries differ considerably in their capacity for formulating and implementing policies, developed countries generally being more able in this respect. Most developing countries lack the human and technical resources required to deal with the full range of their urban development needs. Planning and technical resources are likely to be patchy, and technically competent personnel are often frustrated by organizational barriers and a shortage of resources.

Local constraints may be even greater than those at the national level, as municipal governments may be paralysed by lack of delegation of authority and revenue-raising powers, as well as by a scarcity of skilled human resources and information. Regional mechanisms to harmonize the actions of separate local governments in metropolitan areas are rare. It is not possible to deal with these problems without a major conceptual shift, for a number of reasons:

— The problems of the urban poor are so great and varied that current ways of dealing with them are too slow to be effective. Experience has shown that just doing more of what is being done now will not be enough.

— The changing nature of urban needs makes it dangerous to set out with fixed and preconceived ideas.

— In many countries it is now being recognized that sound urban development is crucial, both for a strong economy and for the well-being of citizens. A strong economy with a sound industrial base is an important goal, but perhaps not the primary one. Health leaders must see that the promotion and protection of health are pursued within the broader framework of urban development, in which health values should be strongly and consistently advocated.

The extent of the conceptual shift needed varies from country to country and city to city according to the current stage of development, the speed of urban growth, and the availability of human and financial resources. It is apparent that everywhere there is a need for the much greater involvement of communities themselves and local authorities in identifying, developing, and implementing the measures necessary for health promotion and protection. The resources needed include not only staff and finance, but also the people, who are the beneficiaries of social development. All agencies and authorities need to act to enable communities and local governments to carry out their obligations to protect the health of the population to the greatest effect. Instead of trying to solve a variety of urban problems themselves, governments will be required to act in an enabling role and facilitate solutions. This implies a degree of decentralization, devolution and power sharing. Urban development can be enhanced if it is closely coordinated with primary health care, with the emphasis on environmental factors in disease prevention and control. Intersectoral coordination needs to be effected at all levels—beginning with the local level, where it is most feasible—to ensure the coherence and effectiveness of policies aimed at improving public health. Women have always had an important role to play in development and health although this is seldom recognized; no attempt at health promotion is likely to be effective unless women's needs, roles, and potential contributions are respected.

In search of solutions

History teaches us that the city is in a good position to mobilize the energy needed to tackle its problems. Many of the factors with a major impact on health are subject to rules, regulations and laws that depend on urban policies. Typical examples are housing, education, water supply, food supply, the prevention of air and water pollution, the control of vectors of transmissible disease, and the development of local transport systems. Together with the health and social services, local cultural attitudes, and levels of employment and income, they largely determine the health status of urban populations.

At the heart of urban policies will always be the popular perception of what the important issues are. It may be possible for external or central directives to influence policy in the short term, but in the longer term what will emerge are policies based on the core values of the local culture. Where there is a local interest in health-related policy, or where such an interest can be brought about by raising awareness, it usually leads to a flowering of different models of effective practice that again depend on the local culture. Health education and health promotion have an important part to play in setting the agenda and raising awareness so that local models of good practice can be developed. One of the advantages of urban areas is usually the presence of highly developed forms of mass communication which can be used to obtain direct access to the population and initiate the kind of debate that is generally needed. Changed expectations about health can only achieve results if they produce greater public participation in the political process and in the fight for health. The mobilization of resources to improve health status will always be associated with the willingness of the public to become involved. In parallel with public participation, the achievement of health for all requires a strengthening of local government. However, it often happens that local government is in need of reform and that the voice of the public as a consumer of public services needs to be louder. This points to the need for political parties, confidential ballots and a choice of candidates.

The poor distribution of insufficient resources is one of the characteristics of underdevelopment, and in urban areas it is possible to find shortages in one place and duplication of services in another. During the past decade, lack of financial resources as a result of the international debt crisis has put a strain on health systems in the developing world. It is becoming clear that the cause lies predominantly in the world financial order rather than the deficiencies of individual countries. Despite every difficulty, health workers struggling against adversity have been responsible for some impressive achievements. For example, as a result of increased immunization coverage and the more effective implementation of oral rehydration therapy, infant mortality rates have decreased in many areas, despite reductions in public health funds. The rapid urbanization now in progress has had many negative effects on health. However, an advantage in the longer term is the stimulus that urbanization gives to planned parenthood with the benefits this brings to families.

We now know that, in the past, many health improvements came about as a result of action outside the medical sector. There is accordingly an unfortunate tendency to present the social and political aspects of health development as being in some way in conflict with the medical and behavioural aspects. In reality this is not the case, particularly as regards the technological advances that offer the possibility of improving the quality of life for those with established disease. From the standpoint of health policy, what is needed is a synthesis and balance between health promotion and

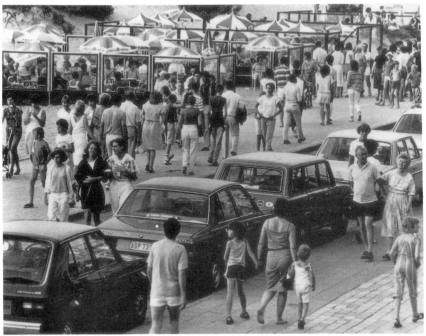

WHO/Zafar (20958)

Enjoying city life: a place to stroll, to relax, to meet, to enjoy a drink with friends.

preventive and curative medical and social care. This can be achieved at city level, given a shared vision of health and a broad political commitment to it.

Key policy issues

- When the health-for-all strategy was first developed there was an assumption that the health problems in rural areas were more urgent than those in the cities. It is now increasingly realized that the rate of growth of urban populations and the conditions under which this growth is occurring make it essential for urgent action to be taken to address the health problems of urban populations.

- Initially it was felt that health for all involved concepts that were of particular relevance to the developing countries. It is now clear that urban populations in industrialized countries can also benefit from policies based on these concepts.

- The effective pursuit of health for all requires sound leadership within communities and the collaboration, on equal terms, of professionals and the public.

- It is essential that all relevant agencies and organizations should collaborate to tackle the urban health problems confronting the world.

- Local government needs to be strong and competent.

- An approach based on health districts and neighbourhood health areas is a powerful tool for ensuring population coverage and an equitable distribution of resources in ways that are compatible with people's needs and expectations.

- There is a need for the development of new health indicators as part of a set of social indicators that can be used to allocate resources and tackle the fundamental causes of urban ill health.

- There has been real progress in moving away from views of health and disease that focus on single causes towards those that acknowledge the multifactorial nature of health and disease. It is now necessary for health institutions to build on this development in the way they operate, in order to promote multidisciplinary and intersectoral action.

Chapter 7
Conclusions

Fundamental challenges in urban health

During the Technical Discussions at the Forty-fourth World Health Assembly, twelve fundamental challenges in the area of urban health were identified:

- population control and environmental sustainability;
- political commitment to urban health;
- decentralization;
- increasing public participation;
- ensuring adequate leadership;
- developing a systematic approach;
- moving towards primary health care;
- obtaining intersectoral collaboration;
- developing a commitment to health promotion;
- ensuring adequate financial resources;
- optimizing the role of nongovernmental, multilateral, and bilateral international agencies;
- establishing city networks for health.

Population and environment

The interaction between urban population growth and environmental degradation is at the heart of the urban health crisis. To reduce urban population growth, effective family planning policies

70

and programmes are required. Policies are needed to raise the status of women and to facilitate family planning as part of a holistic approach to health development, through increased income, better employment, literacy and education (especially of women), better nutrition, access to health services, greater availability of contraceptives, and more effective collaboration between the health system and local populations. Family planning is usually more effective when it is integrated into maternal and child health and primary health care. Population concerns, although varying in magnitude, are similar in developed and developing countries alike. The demographic situation everywhere is a dynamic one and has special implications for health—for example, there is the rapid aging of the population in developed countries and, in contrast, the extreme youthfulness of populations living in the urban areas of the developing world.

Political commitment

An improvement in the health condition of the urban poor will only come about if there is real political commitment to change. This commitment implies a willingness to respond to the will of the people and effect the many changes required in moving from a narrow sectoral policy to one based on a broad view of human and economic development.

Decentralization

It is essential to secure greater local determination and decentralization of power, responsibility, and resources. Care must be taken to ensure that skilled personnel are available at the local level. This approach is important for the development of human resources and of management skills at all levels.

Improved urban health cannot be achieved from the national or even the regional level. Local government needs to participate in policy development by identifying health issues, promoting community involvement, and creating the necessary physical infrastructure. The success of decentralization will depend on the skills and competence of local public health departments. Their needs in training and staff development may have to be met from national or regional resources. If the leadership capacity of municipal health personnel is not supported and developed, health services and their effectiveness will lack credibility in the eyes of the public.

Public participation

It is futile to decide urban health policy without the effective involvement of the public. The most deprived population groups in urban areas are those who are most likely to have weak forms of community organization and whose interests are least likely to be effectively represented. The health sector needs to recognize that its experience and skills in promoting the participation of the public are limited, and that a special effort is needed to reorient and retrain health workers for this important task. Special attention and effort should be devoted to women as the "custodians of family health". Their vulnerability with regard to the impact of urban migration on the family is a matter of particular concern. In both developed and developing cities, the modern universities and hospitals with their high technology often present a stark contrast to the surrounding slums and poor community services. The potential of these institutions to develop and sustain innovative health services should be encouraged.

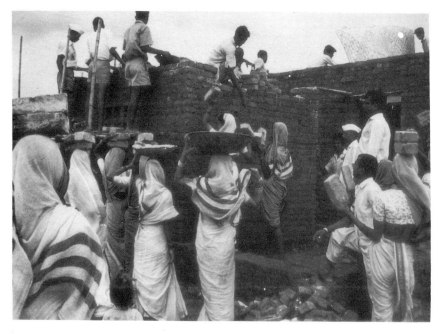

Community participation in slum upgrading efforts can turn poor quality and hazardous houses into dwellings that provide a supportive environment.

Leadership

Effective leadership is needed at all levels within the health sector, but there are obstacles to its achievement. People with appropriate experience and skill are often difficult to hold on to, especially at the municipal level. It may be necessary to offer centrally funded financial inducements for competent people to stay. The health issues raised by urbanization go beyond traditional health concerns, and it is necessary for health workers to act as catalysts for change, working in partnership with a whole range of workers of other types and with the public—the so-called "foreign ministry" role of health workers. For this approach to be successful, attitudes need to be changed and skills increased.

The need for a systematic approach

The need for a systematic approach should not be thwarted by a lack of adequate local data and intelligence. However, most health data originate at the local level and are used in aggregated form at higher administrative levels. There is a need to develop local capacity to collect, manage, and use health data in a systematic way for the planning and evaluation of health services.

Primary health care

Primary health care within district health systems enhances the possibility of mobilizing all the different sectors that influence health in a particular neighbourhood. At its best, this can be a very powerful approach. Furthermore it can serve to direct resources towards local health priorities.

Intersectoral collaboration

Urban development cannot be viewed entirely in terms of either economic objectives or economic indicators. The social and health aspects of the many sectors involved are increasingly being recognized. Information from the various sectors must be brought together to create a holistic view of health and development, and intersectoral action is necessary to ensure that economic development is compatible with health promotion and improvement.

Health promotion

While health promotion and health education in cities remain the responsibility of the health sector, many other sectors are equipped to take part. The whole range of communication resources should be drawn on in providing the public with information about health. Contrary to what many health workers think, the media can be powerful allies in achieving change.

Financial resources

Health should be seen as an investment in the future. However, financial resources are frequently allocated to more conspicuous policy areas, with the result that little money is available for health initiatives. There is a need to adapt taxation systems so that a larger proportion of total revenue comes under the control of the local authorities responsible for health development.

The international debt crisis has had a highly adverse effect on local government in many urban areas. The resolution of many urban health problems is ultimately dependent on the resolution of this crisis. Health promotion and health education should receive priority in funding and there should be special economic incentives to promote investment in disadvantaged urban areas.

The role of nongovernmental organizations and international agencies

For many international agencies, including WHO, the growing urban crisis confirms the importance of many of their programmes of technical cooperation, but also demands significant changes in them. These agencies have successfully identified the global extent of the crisis and how it relates to degradation of the global environment and the overriding issue of sustainable development. Much of the information they provide and the technology they disseminate is directly relevant to the solution of urban problems. Some agencies have successfully fostered an increased interchange of relevant knowledge and experience between countries and cities. Some external support agencies are changing allocation policies towards assigning a greater share of available funds to meeting social development needs—a tendency that should be strengthened.

Apart from better funding from sound urban development, two types of change are now required: first, the widening of technical cooperation to provide better support for national and local efforts and, second, improved internal and interagency coordination of technical cooperation, and external support. Harnessing the potential of nongovernmental, religious, private, and voluntary organizations is a major challenge. By integrating the efforts and resources of these different groups, scarce resources can be used more effectively.

City networks for health

There is clearly a need to promote exchanges of information and experience at the local, national, and international levels, thus making it possible to learn from the failures and successes of both rich and poor countries. Networks such as CITYNET, Metropolis, and WHO's Healthy Cities Project are examples of how this can be done.

It is clear that there has been a significant change in the way in which health is understood. There is now much more awareness of the multifactorial nature of ill health and less of a tendency to look for single causes. There is an increasing realization that all health institutions, including hospitals, should adopt a holistic and integrated approach that will include health promotion as well as treatment and rehabilitation.

WHO continues to play a central role in the development of new ideas and approaches, and is contributing in a decisive way to the task of keeping them abreast of the dynamic changes that are having such a dramatic effect on the health of city-dwellers throughout the world.

References

1. Acheson D. *Public health in England. The report of the Committee of Enquiry into the Future Development of the Public Health Function.* London, Her Majesty's Stationery Office, 1988.

2. McKeown T. *The role of medicine—dream, mirage, or nemesis.* London, Nuffield Provincial Hospitals Trust, 1976.

3. Illich I. *Medical nemesis—the expropriation of health.* Marion Boyars, 1975.

4. Lalonde M. *A new perspective on the health of Canadians.* Ottawa, Ministry of Supply and Services, 1974.

5. The World Commission on Environment and Development. *Our common future.* Oxford, Oxford University Press, 1987.

6. Flynn P. *Ecological models for healthy cities planning. Report on a WHO Workshop, Liverpool, 1988.* Copenhagen, WHO Regional Office for Europe, 1988.

7. WHO/UNICEF. *Primary health care. Report of the International Conference on Primary Health Care, Alma-Ata, USSR, 6–12 September 1978.* Geneva, World Health Organization, 1978 ("Health for All" Series, No. 1).

8. *Global Strategy for Health for All by the Year 2000.* Geneva, World Health Organization, 1981 ("Health for All" Series, No. 3).

9. Finer SE. *The life and times of Sir Edwin Chadwick.* London, Methuen, 1952.

10. *Targets for health for all.* Copenhagen, WHO Regional Office for Europe, 1985.

11. Ashton J, ed. *Healthy cities.* Milton Keynes, Open University Press, 1992.

Selected further reading

Actes du Colloque francophone Villes-santé. Rennes, National School of Public Health, 1990.

Ashton J. Creating a new public health. In: *The new public health in an urban context.* Copenhagen, FADL, 1989 (WHO Healthy Cities Paper, No. 4).

Ashton J. *Healthy cities: action strategies for health promotion.* Liverpool, Department of Public Health, University of Liverpool, 1986.

Ashton J. *Healthy cities—concepts and visions. A resource for the WHO Healthy Cities Project.* Liverpool, Department of Public Health, University of Liverpool, 1988.

Ashton J. Public health and primary care: towards a common agenda. *Public health,* 1990, **104**: 387–398.

Ashton J. Sanitarian becomes ecologist: the new environmental health. *British medical journal,* 1991, **302**: 189–190.

Ashton J. Urban life-style and public health in the city. *The statistician,* 1990, **39**: 147–156.

Ashton J, ed. *Proceedings of the First United Kingdom Healthy Cities Conference, Liverpool, 28–30 March 1988.* Liverpool, Department of Public Health, University of Liverpool, 1990.

Ashton J, Seymour H. *The new public health.* Milton Keynes, Open University Press, 1988.

Ashton J, Ubido J. The healthy city and the ecological idea. Paper presented at the Society for the Social History of Medicine. *Social history of medicine,* 1991, **4**(1): 173–181.

Ashton J et al. Healthy cities: WHO's new public health initiative. *Health promotion,* 1986, **1**: 319–323.

Ashton J et al. Promoting the new public health in one region. *Health education journal,* 1986, **45**(3): 174–179.

Ashton JR. *Esmedune 2000. A healthy Liverpool (vision or dream).* Liverpool, Department of Community Health, University of Liverpool, 1988.

Basta SS. Nutrition and health in low income urban areas of the Third World. *Ecology of food and nutrition,* 1977, **6**: 113–124.

Beyond health care. Proceedings of a Working Conference on Healthy Public Policy. *Canadian journal of public health*, 1985, **76** (suppl): 1–104.

Bradley D et al. *Relative health impacts of environmental health problems in urban areas of developing countries*. London, London School of Hygiene and Tropical Medicine, 1990 (report submitted to the World Bank).

Brown V. *Social health in a small city*. Paper presented to the 12th World Conference on Health Education, Dublin, September 1985. Canberra, Health Promotion Branch, Australian Capital Territory Health Authority, 1985.

Chabot JHT. The Chinese system of health care. *Tropical and geographical medicine*, 1976, **28**: 87–134.

Chadwick E. *Report on the sanitary condition of the labouring population of Great Britain* [1842]. Edinburgh, Edinburgh University Press, 1965.

Chave S. *Recalling the Medical Officer of Health*. London, King Edward's Hospital Fund, 1987.

Cointreau SJ. *Environmental management of urban solid wastes in developing countries: a project guide*. Washington, DC, World Bank, 1982 (World Bank Technical Paper, No. 5).

Duhl L. The healthy city: its function and its future. *Health promotion*, 1986, **1**: 55–60.

Ghosh SJ et al. Mortality patterns in an urban birth cohort. *Indian journal of medical research*, 1979, **69**: 616–623.

Giroult E. Transports ou santé: faut-il choisir? [Transport or health: must we choose?] *Cahiers du génie urbain*, 1992, No. 4.

Global strategy for shelter to the year 2000. Nairobi, United Nations Centre for Human Settlements (Habitat), 1990.

Guenot C, Gueguer R. *Les indicateurs de santé dans la ville*. [Health indicators in the town.] Nancy, 1992.

Hancock T. Lalonde and beyond: looking back at "A new perspective on the health of Canadians". *Health promotion*, 1986 **1**(1): 93–100

Hancock T. Healthy Toronto—a vision of a healthy city. In: *Healthy cities— concepts and visions. A resource for the WHO Healthy Cities project*. Liverpool, Department of Community Health, University of Liverpool, 1988.

Hardoy JE et al., ed. *The poor die young: housing and health in Third World cities*. London, Earthscan Publications, 1990.

Hardoy JE, Satterthwaite D. *Squatter citizen: life in the urban Third World*. London, Earthscan Publications, 1989.

Harpham T et al., ed. *In the shadow of the city: community health and the urban poor*. Oxford, Oxford University Press, 1988.

Hauser PM et al. *Population and the urban future*. New York, State University of New York Press, 1982.

Health of Towns Commission. *Remedial measures, local reports*, 2nd report, vol. 1. London, William Clowes and Son, 1845.

Henri A. *Environments and happenings*. London, Thames and Hudson, 1974.

Lacombe R, Poirier L. Villes et villages en santé. [Towns and villages in health.] *Santé, société,* 1991, **13** (3–4).

Lewis RA. *Edwin Chadwick and the public health movement, 1832–1854.* London, Longmans Green and Co, 1952.

Liverpool City Planning Department. *Social area study. The results in brief.* Liverpool, 1984.

Liverpool City Planning Department. *Inequalities in health in Liverpool.* Liverpool, 1986.

Lovelock J. *The age of Gaia—a biography of our living earth.* Oxford, Oxford University Press, 1989.

Mayor's Survey. *KIDSPLACE—technical report.* Seattle, WA, 1984.

Milio N. *Promoting health through public policy.* Ottawa, Canadian Public Health Association, 1986.

Oberoi AS. Urban population growth, employment and poverty in developing countries: a conceptual framework for policy analysis In: *Consequences of rapid population growth in developing countries.* New York, United Nations, Department of International Economic and Social Affairs, 1989 (ESA/P/WP.110), pp. 287–331.

O'Neill P. *Health crisis 2000.* Copenhagen, WHO Regional Office for Europe, 1983.

Ottawa Charter for Health Promotion. *Health promotion,* 1986, **1**(4): iii–v.

Patchwork in urban health care. Papers from the Kellogg International Fellowship Program in Health. Michigan State University, 1990.

Rapport final du Deuxième Congrès inter-regional villes-santé en langue française. Montpellier, 1991.[1]

Report of the Interregional Meeting on City Health: the challenge of social justice. Karachi, 27–30 November 1989. Geneva, World Health Organization, 1990 (unpublished document WHO/SHS/NHP/90.3; available on request from Strengthening of Health Services, World Health Organization, 1211 Geneva 27, Switzerland).

Rochon J. *Rapport de la Commission d'Enquête sur les services de santé et les services sociaux. [Report of the Commission of Inquiry on the health and social services.]* Montreal, Publications du Quebec, 1988.

Romieu I et al. Urban air pollution in Latin America and the Caribbean: health perspectives. *World health statistics quarterly,* 1990, **43**(3): 153–167.

Sabouraud A. *Le réseau français des villes-santé.* Rennes, 1992.[1]

Sadik N. *Remembering youth worldwide: the global impact of too early child bearing.* Speech delivered at the Tenth Anniversary Conference of the Center for Population Options. Washington, DC, 1990.

Smith C. *Community-based health initiatives. A handbook for voluntary groups.* London, National Council of Voluntary Organizations, 1982.

---

[1]Available from Environmental Health in Rural and Urban Development and Housing, World Health Organization, 1211 Geneva 27, Switzerland.

Stolnitz GA. *Urbanization and rural-to-urban migration in relation to LDC fertility.* Bloomington, University of Indiana, 1984.

Tabibzadeh I et al. *Spotlight on the cities: improving urban health in developing countries.* Geneva, World Health Organization, 1989.

United Nations Centre for Human Settlements (Habitat). *Urbanization and sustainable development in the Third World: an unrecognized global issue.* Nairobi, 1989.

United Nations. Department of International Economic and Social Affairs. *Results of the sixth population inquiry among governments.* New York, 1990 (ST/ESA/SER.R/104), pp. 24 and 49.

United Nations. Department of International Economic and Social Affairs. *The sex and age distribution of population.* New York, 1991 (ST/ESA/SER.A/122).

United Nations. Department of International Economic and Social Affairs. *World population prospects 1990.* New York, 1990 (ST/ESA/SER.A/120).

United Nations Fund for Population Activities. *State of world population: UNFPA annual report, 1985.* New York, United Nations, 1986.

Villes et santé. [Towns and health.] Rennes, National School of Public Health, 1990.

Vuori H. Primary health care in Europe: problems and solutions. *Community medicine,* 1984, **6**: 221–231.

White BD. *History of the Corporation of Liverpool.* Liverpool, Liverpool University Press, 1951.

WHO Regional Office for Europe. *European Charter on Environment and Health.* Copenhagen, 1988.

WHO Regional Office for Europe. *Healthy cities—action strategies for health promotion.* Copenhagen, 1986.

World Health Organization. *Urbanization and its implications for child health: potential for action.* Geneva, 1989.

World Health Organization. *Environmental health in urban development: report of a WHO Expert Committee.* Geneva, 1991 (WHO Technical Report Series, No. 807).

Wohl AS. *Endangered lives. Public health in Victorian Britain.* London, Methuen, 1984.

World Bank. *World developement report 1990.* Oxford, Oxford University Press, 1990.